Plaque and Calculus Removal

Plaque and Calculus Removal

Considerations for the Professional

David L. Cochran, DDS, PhD, MS, MMSci
Professor and Chairman
Department of Periodontics
The University of Texas Health Science Center
San Antonio, Texas

Kenneth L. Kalkwarf, DDS, MS
Professor and Dean, Dental School
The University of Texas Health Science Center
San Antonio, Texas

Michael A. Brunsvold, DDS, MS
Associate Professor
Department of Periodontics
The University of Texas Health Science Center
San Antonio, Texas

with **Carol Brooks,** RDH
School of Dentistry
Medical College of Virginia
Richmond, Virginia

quintessence
books

Quintessence Publishing Co, Inc
Chicago, Berlin, London, Tokyo, Moscow, Prague, Sofia, and Warsaw

Library of Congress Cataloging-In-Publication Data

Cochran, David L. (David Lee), 1952-
    Plaque and calculus removal: considerations for the professional
/David L. Cochran, Kenneth L. Kalkwarf, Michael A. Brunsvold:
with Carol Brooks.
        p.   cm.
    Includes bibliographical references and index.
    ISBN 0-86715-285-0
    1. Dental prophylaxis. 2. Dental plaque. 3. Dental calculus.
I. Kalkwarf, Kenneth L. II. Brunsvold, Michael A. III. Brooks, Carol.
IV. Title.
    [DNLM: 1. Dental Prophylaxis—methods. 2. Dental Deposits—therapy
3. Dental Prophylaxis—instrumentation
WU 113 C663p 1994]
RK60.7.C63 1994
617.6'01—dc20
DNLM/DLC
for Library of Congress   94-17876
                                                               CIP

Editor: Patricia Bereck Weikersheimer
Designer: Jennifer Ann Sabella

Printed in Hong Kong

Contents

Preface ix

1 Rationale for Plaque and Calculus Removal 1

Plaque **1**
   Significance of Plaque **1**
   Plaque Formation **4**
   Bacterial Composition **5**
   Dental Stains **5**
   Plaque Removal **6**
Calculus **6**
   Scaling/Root Planing **7**
   Closed/Open Scaling and Root Planing **9**

2 Mechanical Removal of Plaque and Calculus by the Patient 13

Toothbrushes **15**
Brushing Techniques **17**
Other Toothbrushing Considerations **19**
Interdental Cleansing **21**

Interdental Devices 22
   Dental Floss 22
   Flossing Techniques 27
Interdental Brushes 28
Single-tufted Brushes 30
Other Mechanical Aids 31
   Irrigators 33
   Abrasives 35
   Additional Devices 36

3   Mechanical Removal of Plaque and Calculus by the Professional 39

Mechanical Instrumentation 39
Electronic Instrumentation 42
Abrasives 42
Calculus Removal 43
   Evaluation 43
   Pain Control 45
Pre-instrumentation Rinsing 47
Instrumentation 48
   Hand/Mechanical Instruments 54
   Limitations of Hand/Mechanical Instrumentation 54
Adjuncts for Professional Calculus Removal 56
   Magnification 56
   Illumination 56
   Papillae Reflection 57
   Root Sensitivity 58
Scaling/Root Planing for Special Patients 59
   Cardiac Considerations 59
   Infectious Diseases 60

4   Powered Instruments 61

Ultrasonic Instuments 62
   Mechanism of Action 62
   Indications and Limitations 62
   Guidelines for Use 63
   Effects on Teeth and Other Oral Tissues 64
   Comparison of Ultrasonics to Hand Instruments 65

Modified Ultrasonic Instruments 65
Sonic Instruments 67
Air Polishing Devices 68
Rotating Instruments 69

5 Maintenance of Instruments 73

Sharpening Rationale 73
Sharpening Techniques 75
Sterilization 76

6 Chemotherapeutic Removal of Plaque and Calculus 81

Chlorhexidine 82
Essential Oils 83
Non-ADA Approved Agents 84
  Stannous Fluoride 84
  Sanguinarine 84
  Oxygenating Agents 85
  Prebrushing Rinse 85
  Quaternary Ammonium Compounds 86

7 Implant Considerations 89

Implants and Oral Hygiene 90
Plaque Removal on Implant Surfaces 90

Index 99

Preface

This book addresses the removal of plaque and calculus from teeth and implants, presenting procedures for both the patient and the professional to perform. Special consideration is given to the removal of plaque and calculus around endosseous dental implants.

This book is written primarily to assist the general dentist and hygienist in understanding various consequences of plaque accumulation and what is required to remove plaque and its calcified product, calculus. It is not intended to be a comprehensive review of plaque and calculus nor to describe specific mechanical aspects of removal techniques. Several excellent texts and manuals on each of these topics already exist. This book should provide supplemental material to the more detailed texts and help the reader assimilate various considerations for plaque and calculus removal.

An overview of the significance of plaque and calculus formation is given as is the biologic rationale for their removal. It is important to note that plaque is recognized as the etiologic agent for gingivitis and that it is a necessary, but not always sufficient, etiologic agent for periodontitis. Other factors play a role in the loss of connective tissue and clearly many of these factors involve the host response. This book does not contain in-depth discussions of these etiologic aspects of periodontal diseases or the potential pathogenetic aspects of the diseases. The reader is referred to texts on periodontal diseases for this information.

Many studies conclude that the critical component for successful periodontal therapy lies in the maintenance of a relatively plaque-free environment. Furthermore, long-term studies have shown that the specific type of periodontal therapy administered is not critical if good plaque control is consistently obtained. Because it is absolutely essential that the patient with periodontal disease removes plaque daily, this book provides a discussion on techniques for plaque removal by patients. Specific procedures are described, as are the advantages and disadvantages of some currently available products touted for daily plaque removal.

Information is also provided on the removal of plaque and calculus by the dental professional, including both traditional mechanical and electronically assisted procedures. Many practitioners have developed variations on specific techniques, several of which are discussed. Specific adjuncts that are helpful in the removal of plaque and calculus are also presented, in addition to procedures used to properly maintain hand instruments.

[1]

Rationale for Plaque and Calculus Removal

Plaque

Significance of Plaque

The periodontal diseases can be classified into two broad categories: gingivitis and periodontitis. Gingivitis is defined as inflammation of the gingiva and is a reversible condition. Many forms of periodontitis probably exist but the definition of this disease can be considered as inflammation of the periodontal tissues and loss of connective tissue.[1] The etiologic agent for gingivitis was examined in the classic work by Löe et al.[2] In these longitudinal studies, dental students were examined and their teeth cleaned so that the gingival tissues were as plaque-free as possible and non-inflamed, ie, pink, healthy, had normal contours and did not bleed following gingival probing (Fig 1-1). At that time all oral hygiene procedures were discontinued and plaque was allowed to accumulate for up to 4 weeks. Gingivitis developed within 21 days in all subjects (Fig 1-2). The subjects then underwent a professional tooth cleaning and oral hygiene procedures were instituted. Within 14 days after plaque removal, all gingival tissues returned to a healthy state. This experiment has been repeated a number of times, always with the same result. Thus, a very strong cause-and-effect relationship is known for plaque accumulation and the development of gingivitis (Figs 1-3 and 1-4). The relationship between plaque accumulation and gingivitis provides the foundation for plaque removal procedures by the professional and by the patient as the primary procedure to prevent or treat gingivitis.

Much less is known about the etiologic factors of periodontitis. It appears that plaque is required for disease initiation, but it alone is not sufficient to cause the disease. An epidemiologic study of periodontitis in a population of individuals who had never been exposed to dental care was performed by Löe et al.[3] The results showed that approximately 8% of the population had very severe periodontitis while 81% had moderate periodontitis. The most surprising finding was that approximately 11% of the population, despite very large amounts of plaque and calculus, did not show signs of periodontitis. This study demonstrates that plaque alone is not sufficient to cause periodontitis. It is now apparent that the interaction between host response and plaque is critical for the initiation and progression of periodontitis. It is obvious from these studies, however, that plaque is required for the initiation of the periodontal diseases. Thus, preventive therapies for periodontal diseases should always include the removal of plaque.

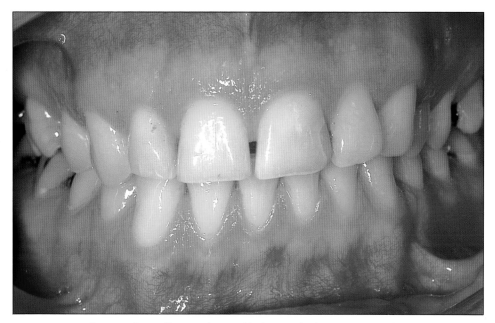

Fig 1-1. Facial view of maxillary and mandibular teeth showing normal contours, noninflamed gingiva, and pink, healthy tissues.

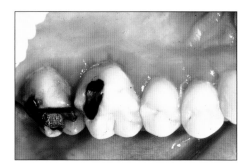

Fig 1-2. Lingual view of left maxillary posterior teeth and gingiva. Marginal and interproximal tissue is red, swollen, and severely inflamed, indicative of gingivitis.

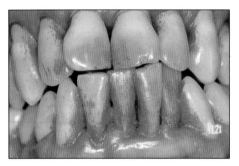

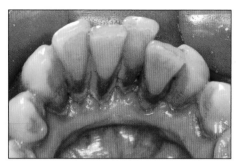

Fig 1-3. Anterior view of periodontally involved teeth stained with disclosing solution. The plaque is visualized as red stain.

Fig 1-4. Lingual view of mandibular anterior teeth. Plaque is stained red with disclosing solution. Calculus is observed on the interproximal surfaces below the cementoenamel junctions.

Plaque Formation

The formation of dental plaque begins with the deposition of an organic layer called the dental pellicle on the tooth surface. The thickness of the pellicle usually ranges from 1 to 2 µm and forms within a couple hours on a cleaned tooth surface. Grant, Stern, and Listgarten[4] have described deposition of the pellicle in four stages: *1)* bathing of the tooth surfaces by salivary fluids, which contain numerous protein constituents; *2)* selective adsorption of certain negatively and positively charged glycoproteins; *3)* surface denaturation and acid precipitation resulting in loss of solubility of the adsorbed proteins; and *4)* alteration of the glycoproteins by enzymes from bacteria and the oral secretions. Once formed, the dental pellicle is actively involved in bacterial colonization. Protein-protein and protein-carbohydrate interactions occur and provide receptors for adhesions or other binding proteins. Specific proteins present in the pellicle then selectively bind certain bacterial species. After the initial layer of bacteria attaches to the pellicle, many different bacterial species rapidly accumulate and the composition of the bacterial flora begins to change. As maturation of the plaque occurs, salivary components continue to play a role. Proteins and adherence factors bind to the developing matrix and intercellular bacterial adhesion occurs.

Bacterial Composition

The composition of dental plaque varies among individuals and is dependent on the specific tooth surface. The appearance is definite, with bacterial cells arranged as colonies in clumps or columns. Various gram-positive species, including streptococci, form a predominant part of the newly formed supragingival deposit. As plaque matures, facultative microorganisms proliferate, creating an environment with low oxygen tension and the growth of anaerobic microorganisms. In subgingival areas, motile, gram-negative rods and spirochetes predominate. These bacteria are often arranged in zones or layers with adherent layers near the tooth surface and more loosely arranged layers closer to the tissue. Studies on the bacterial composition of healthy and diseased gingiva have now been documented. Coccoid and short rod forms are associated with healthy gingiva. Distinctly different bacterial floras are associated with different forms of periodontitis.

Dental Stains

Staining of adherent tooth deposits can range from light to severe and take on a variety of forms. The staining constitutes an esthetic problem but contributes little to the pathogenesis of disease. Food stains by various pigments such as those in tea and coffee, as well as by tobacco tar, make up a large part of the stain normally encountered. Staining by bacteria also occurs and can range from brown and black to green and orange. Recently, brown staining by antimicrobial mouth-rinses has been commonly found. Staining from this source can become so prominent that compliance with use of the antimicrobial mouthwash is precluded.

Plaque Removal

As previously noted, dental plaque is associated with both gingivitis and periodontitis. Plaque removal thus constitutes an essential component of the therapeutic approach to preventing and controlling these diseases. Plaque removal can be accomplished by the professional, the patient, or both. After a tooth surface has been cleaned and the plaque removed, new dental pellicle is deposited very rapidly (within minutes to hours). Frequent removal of plaque results in the occurrence of less mature forms of dental plaque, which contain fewer numbers of the potentially pathogenic bacterial colonies. Subgingival bacteria are also affected by daily supragingival plaque control. Thus, effective removal of plaque is a desirable goal for the prevention of the periodontal diseases. Plaque accumulation occurs predominantly in areas protected against friction from food, cheeks, tongue, and lips. Prime locations for plaque deposits are at the gingival margin and in the gingival crevice. Many studies indicate that plaque removal by both the professional and the patient at very frequent intervals is the most effective way to control periodontal diseases.

Calculus

While plaque and the bacteria associated with plaque have been implicated as the primary etiologic agents for gingivitis and periodontitis, maturation and calcification of plaque into dental calculus is also a primary concern for the dental therapist. Calculus deposits harbor bacteria from the patient's mechanical and chemical cleansing approaches[5] and provide an environment conducive to continued bacterial growth. Removal of calculus deposits should be a primary goal for the therapist involved in treating periodontal diseases.

Exposure of bacterial plaque to tissue fluid (saliva or crevicular fluid) will result in mineralization of the plaque and formation of calculus. Calculus deposits are classified according to their physical location. Supragingival calculus attaches to the tooth's surface coronal to the gingival margin and subgingival calculus forms apical to the gingival margin. Supragingival calculus is usually chalky in appearance and relatively easy to remove compared to the dark brown or black subgingival calculus deposits. Removal of both types of calculus eliminates the nidus of resident bacteria in the calculus mass and allows the patient access for removal of bacterial plaque from the tooth's surface.

Scaling/Root Planing

Scaling is defined as the removal of calculus from the surfaces of teeth, while *root planing* may be described as smoothing of the root surfaces.[1] Root planing includes the removal of rough cementum or dentin that is impregnated with calculus (Fig 1-5). Scaling and root planing are usually performed together as a therapeutic approach for gingivitis and periodontitis.

Traditionally, the end points of scaling/root planing have been the inability of the clinician to mechanically or visibly detect remaining calculus and the perception of a smooth root surface. Obviously, these end points are subjective.

Numerous studies have confirmed the inability of clinicians to remove subgingival calculus deposits with traditional scaling and root planing procedures (Fig 1-6).[6] However, in many cases, a positive healing response of the periodon-

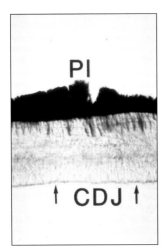

Fig 1-5. Micrograph demonstrating plaque penetrating into the superficial layers of cementum on the tooth root. CDJ and arrows represent the cementodentinal junction; Pl, plaque.

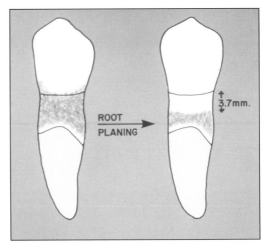

Fig 1-6. Shown is the area of the tooth root accessible to closed root planing procedures.

tium occurs despite the fact that calculus deposits undoubtedly remain.[7] Robertson[8] probably best explains the situation when he states, "while total elimination of etiologic factors is the appropriate treatment goal, reduction of plaque and calculus below the threshold level that is acceptable to the host appears to control the infection process and improve the clinical signs of inflammation."

Based on this hypothesis, the therapeutic end points for scaling/root planing should not be the inability to detect calculus deposits or the perception of a smooth root surface. The clinician must instead evaluate the healing response of the periodontal tissues following completion of therapy. If tissue healing progresses to completion with no remaining signs of inflammation, one has achieved a successful end point. If signs of inflammation remain, additional treatment is indicated.

Closed/Open Scaling and Root Planing

Many approaches have been advocated for the removal of calculus from the tooth surface. Each approach will be described in more detail later in this text. Supragingival approaches are all relatively straightforward unless gingival contours are unusual (Figs 1-7 and 1-8), with the deposits visibly identified and removal procedures easily controlled. The response of the marginal tissues during healing after treatment is easily evaluated.

Appropriate methods to remove subgingival calculus are much more controversial. The primary discussions revolve around the appropriate type of instrument (hand/mechanical vs powered) and whether the procedure should be accomplished with a closed approach (inserting the instrument into the gingival crevice and working by tactile sense) or with an open approach where the gingival tissue is surgically reflected, allowing instrumentation and evaluation with direct visual guidance.

A closed approach is advantageous in that it is not as time-consuming (it does not require tissue incision, tissue reflection, suturing, and subsequent postsurgical follow-up).

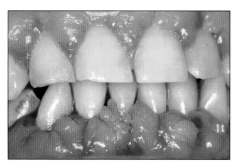

Fig 1-7. Facial view of maxillary and mandibular anterior teeth of a patient taking cyclosporin.

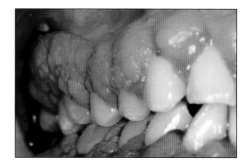

Fig 1-8. Right posterior facial view of same patient as seen in Fig 1-7 demonstrating the extreme gingival contours that can occur in certain patients taking particular medications. These contours complicate plaque removal procedures.

Closed scaling and root planing may be performed by a dental hygienist, potentially controlling the cost of treatment.

Many clinicians argue that an open approach to scaling and root planing is more efficacious because it allows better control of instrumentation and direct visualization of the calculus deposits. Many clinicians believe that these advantages far outweigh the extra steps involved in delivering an open approach and the fact that therapy involving tissue incisions and reflection may not be legally delivered by an auxiliary dental care provider.

Results of controlled studies have confirmed that open procedures are more effective than closed procedures in the removal of calculus deposits.[9,10] The effectiveness of open procedures over closed procedures increases as the depth of periodontal pockets and related subgingival calculus deposits becomes deeper. Recent studies have confirmed that total subgingival calculus removal is rare regardless of whether the therapeutic approach is closed or open.

Based on the results of controlled, longitudinal therapy trials,[11,12] the most prudent approach to calculus removal is to initially perform scaling and root planing procedures with a closed approach. This allows the procedure to be performed in an efficacious manner, without exposing the patient to a surgical procedure, and allows therapy to be performed by either a dentist or dental hygienist. As previously described, outcome assessment following instrumentation should be by post-therapy evaluation of the inflammatory response in the periodontal tissues. Additional instrumentation with an open approach is appropriate at those sites that do not completely respond to closed scaling and root planing.

This sequencing of therapy allows all sites capable of responding to the closed approach the chance to respond. More aggressive and costly therapy, involving surgical tissue reflection, suturing, and more rigorous follow-up, is confined to sites that do not respond adequately to closed instrumentation.

The sequencing of therapy for individuals with chronic, inflammatory periodontal diseases should be:

1. Initiation of a personal oral hygiene program to allow the patient to effectively and efficiently disorganize accumulations of bacterial plaque on a daily basis.

2. Re-evaluation of tissue response following a period of at least 7 to 14 days of effective personal plaque removal. If tissues remain inflamed, and it is suspected that calculus is playing a role in the cause of the inflammation, closed scaling/root planing procedures should be initiated. An attempt to remove all supragingival and subgingival deposits should be made. For patient comfort and convenience, treatment may involve one or more appointments and may require the use of analgesics or anesthetic agents.

3. Evaluation of tissue response should be repeated after allowing sufficient time for tissue healing (6 to 8 weeks). If specific sites have not responded and inflammation remains, they should be targeted for more aggressive therapy involving surgical reflection of tissues to allow open instrumentation.

4. Successful elimination of inflammation should be followed by the establishment of an appropriate program of supportive periodontal maintenance allowing periodic professional monitoring of periodontal health and appropriate supplemental therapy.

References

1. Glossary of Periodontal Terms, ed 3. The American Academy of Periodontology, 1992.
2. Löe H, Theilade E, Jensen SB. Experimental gingivitis in man. J Periodontol 1965;36:177.
3. Löe H, Anerud A, Boysen H, Morrison E. Natural history of periodontal disease in man. J Clin Periodontol 1986;13:431.

4. Grant DA, Stern IB, Listgarten MA (eds): Microbiology (plaque). In Periodontics, ed 6. St Louis: CV Mosby Co; 1988:147.

5. Schwartz JP, Rateitschak-Plüss EM, Guggenheim R, Düggelin M, Rateitschak KH. Effectiveness of open flap root debridement with rubber cups, interdental plastic tips and prophy paste. An SEM study. J Clin Periodontol 1993;20:1-6.

6. Sherman PR, Hutchens LH, Jewson LG. The effectiveness of subgingival scaling and root planing. II. Clinical responses related to residual calculus. J Periodontol 1990;61:9-15.

7. Kaldahl W, Kalkwarf K, Patil K, et al. Evaluation of four modalities of periodontal therapy. J Periodontol 1988;59:783.

8. Robertson PB. The residual calculus paradox. J Periodontol 1990;61:65-66.

9. Brayer WK, Mellonig JT, Dunlap RM, Marinak KW, Carson RE. Scaling and root planing effectiveness: The effect of root surface access and operator experience. J Periodontol 1989;60:67-72.

10. Parashis AO, Anagnou-Varelzides A, Demetriou N. Calculus removal from multirooted teeth with and without surgical access. J Clin Periodontol 1993;20:63-68.

11. Pihlstrom B, McHugh R, Oliphant T, Ortiz-Campos C. Comparison of surgical and non-surgical treatment of periodontal disease. J Clin Periodontol 1983;10:524.

12. Ramfjord S, Caffesse R, Morrison E. Four modalities of periodontal therapy compared over five years. J Periodont Res 1987;22:222.

[2]

Mechanical Removal of Plaque and Calculus by the Patient

One of the most critical aspects of successful plaque removal and disease control is comprehension by the patient of the role of plaque and, equally important, its appearance. Educating the patient on the clinical appearance and location of plaque is as essential to preventing and treating periodontal diseases as the mechanical or chemical debridement techniques the patient uses. It is also important for the patient to understand the relationship of bleeding gums and periodontal diseases—being able to visualize the target of plaque control efforts will give direction to those efforts.

To the uneducated or uninspired patient, the concept of plaque accumulation is difficult to comprehend. These patients may brush their teeth without comprehending the goal of their plaque control efforts. They may not even know how healthy tissue or a clean mouth feels. This is in contrast to the motivated patient, who has knowledge of the structures of the mouth and can identify difficult areas where supragingival plaque accumulation may be a problem.

Initially, patients may be unable to visualize plaque accumulation on their teeth without the aid of special dyes. The use of plaque disclosants will enable the patient to determine the effectiveness of their plaque control, illustrating how much plaque is on the teeth and where it is located (see Figs 1-3 and 1-4). When this is done at the beginning of oral hygiene instruction, it provides the patient and clinician with a baseline from which to evaluate the success of future plaque control efforts. Several commercial products are available that stain supragingival plaque and render it visible. Colored dyes stain plaque red but are often times unacceptable to patients since they also stain the lips, gingiva and other oral tissues for several hours. Also available are relatively colorless fluorescein dyes, which make plaque visible when illuminated with blue-filtered light. These may be less objectionable to some patients.

These dyes can be routinely used by the patient to evaluate the thoroughness of their home care efforts. At subsequent dental appointments, supragingival plaque control effectiveness can be measured and compared to baseline and techniques adjusted as indicated.

Before beginning a discussion of the various dental devices recommended by clinicians and used by patients to perform tooth cleaning, it is necessary to establish a basic premise. This premise is that the devices and methods recommended must be individually adapted to specific patient needs. These needs vary depending on tooth positioning, gingival contours, embrasure size, tissue health, patient dexterity, and patient motivation. It is also necessary to establish that a patient's home care routine, tailored to his specific needs, is not a static program. Rather, it is a regimen that evolves with time as varying aspects of oral hygiene are presented, mastered, assessed, and readapted to changing needs. This approach requires a long-term commitment to care by both the clinician and the patient.

Gone are the days when the dental professional can give patients a toothbrush, floss, and manufacturer's brochure and expect them to be responsible for their oral hygiene. In place of this scenario, the dental professional has been inundated by oral hygiene products and dental devices, making the decision of what to recommend to patients difficult. Also, while it is often advantageous to have a patient use several different devices to meet his or her specific oral hygiene needs, few patients can assimilate the instructions, recommendations, and adaptations necessary to master all appropriate techniques in one appointment. This again indicates the need for a long-term strategy and a continuing commitment to oral health.

Toothbrushes

Toothbrushing is the most commonly used mechanical method to remove supragingival plaque from the occlusal surfaces and broad, flat tooth contours. However, the average person removes only about 50% of the plaque present when brushing their teeth.[1] In efforts to improve this, various evaluations of the composition, size, and shape of toothbrushes and their filaments have been conducted. It has been found that certain standard criteria are present in an effective toothbrush. These are soft bristles, a multitufted head, and end-rounded filaments. Research has found that soft, nylon, multitufted bristles removed more plaque than hard bristles, even when applying less pressure. It has also been noted that brushes that have end-rounded filaments produce less gingival abrasion than filaments cut straight across.[2]

Until recently, the most common brush design has been flat plane bristles (Fig 2-1). In contrast, an alternative design with a rippled bristle pattern has been recently introduced that may increase the efficiency of plaque removal in interproximal areas (Fig 2-2).

Other parts of a toothbrush may display various designs. These include the shape, angulation, length, and diameter of the head, shank, and handle (Figs 2-3 and 2-4). Although these variations may have less of a direct impact on plaque removal and tissue health, they may influence a patient's ability to control the brush and adapt it within their mouth. Patient needs and preferences determine which brush is best for an individual. This may necessitate the need for more than one type of brush, depending on difficult-to-reach areas or specific periodontal conditions.

Timing of toothbrush replacement generally depends on the condition of the brush. Splaying and matting of bristles indicate the need for replacement. Brushing habits and storage influence toothbrush longevity. In an effort to establish a guideline, it is recommended that toothbrushes be replaced every 3 months to maintain optimal cleaning ability.

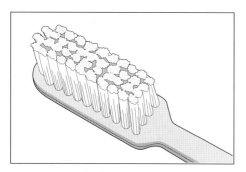

Fig 2-1. Head of toothbrush demonstrating a flat plane of bristles.

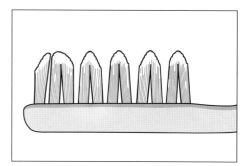

Fig 2-2. A toothbrush head with a rippled bristle pattern designed to facilitate interproximal cleaning.

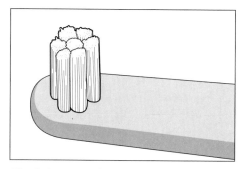

Fig 2-3. An end-tufted brush with a flat plane of bristles.

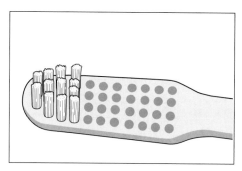

Fig 2-4. Head of a toothbrush that has been modified to reach specific areas of the teeth and gums.

Brushing Techniques

A number of toothbrush techniques have been described in the literature, including horizontal strokes, vertical strokes, roll technique, circular brushing, scrub techniques, and vibratory techniques. These techniques can be a source of frustration for patients as they receive frequently changing recommendations for brushing methods, depending on the clinician. Despite the fact that certain techniques may be more appropriate for certain situations, or easier for certain individuals to perform, no single method has been shown to be clinically superior. The basis of most techniques is directional motion, with placement and angulation of the bristles in relation to the tooth and the gingiva. Plaque removal by toothbrushing is dependent on the refinement of these motions, their duration and frequency, and the type of brush used. Correct and conscientious application of these motions results in successful plaque removal.

Of these several methods available, the Bass technique, with certain modifications, is generally considered the method of choice, especially for plaque removal along the gingival margin. The Bass technique calls for the bristles of a soft, multitufted toothbrush to be placed at the gingival margin, angled toward the soft tissue, generally at a 45-degree angle to the long axis of the tooth (Figs 2-5 and 2-6). Light pressure is applied, and the bristles are worked into the crevicular and interproximal regions with a vibratory, circular motion. This allows the bristles to cleanse the gingival margin and even advance slightly subgingivally. The cleansing area is the length of the head of the toothbrush. Overlapping strokes are applied so that all areas of the dentition are reached. A modification that can be applied involves the additional step of sweeping the bristles occlusally following the vibratory motion. This action ensures complete cleansing of the facial and lingual surfaces. Back-and-forth horizontal strokes are used to brush the occlusal surfaces.[1]

As an alternative to manual brushing, several types of electric toothbrushes have been developed. These are especially useful to those patients who have dexterity or mastery problems with a manual brush or who are unable to relinquish a destructive or ineffective stroke. Brushing motions include one or a combination of the following actions: reciprocating (back and forth), orbital (circular), accurate (up and down), vibratory and rotating tufts of bristles that continually reverse directions. Even with these varying motions, effectiveness still depends on brush and bristle placement.

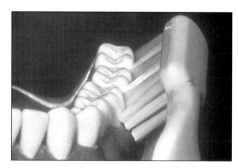

Fig 2-5. Demonstration of a soft-bristled brush at a 45-degree angle to the teeth at the gingival margin showing toothbrush placement in the Bass brushing technique.

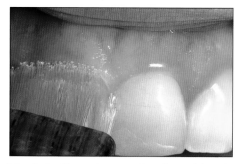

Fig 2-6. Clinical example of toothbrush placement during the Bass brushing technique.

Other Toothbrushing Considerations

Two important considerations that determine the effectiveness of toothbrushing, both manual and electric, as an oral hygiene measure are sequential brushing technique and time spent brushing. Sequential brushing enables the patient to keep track of areas brushed, aids in toothbrushing habit formation, and ensures that all areas are reached. Even with the best brush and best method, effectiveness is difficult to achieve if adequate time is not spent brushing. In industrialized countries, the average person brushes once daily. Typically, when their brushing habits are observed, people brush from 33 seconds to 2 minutes.[3] It is estimated that unobserved brushers probably spend even less time. Inappropriate sequencing or inadequate time result in areas missed, usually at the gingival margin, and particularly on the proximal and lingual surfaces of teeth. Complete removal of all reachable plaque remains the goal of effective plaque control and disease prevention.

Patients who use a toothbrush with hard bristles, incorrect bristle angulation or placement, too long or vigorous a brushing stroke, or extremely abrasive toothpaste may cause acute or chronic tissue problems. Acute soft tissue trauma can appear as reddened, denuded, or ulcerated areas (Fig 2-7). Chronic soft tissue trauma can result in gingival recession, rolled marginal gingiva, or gingival clefting (Fig 2-8). Tooth surface alterations as a result of chronic toothbrush trauma include wedge-shaped grooves. Hard and soft tissue trauma occurs most frequently at the cementoenamel junction area on the facial surfaces of premolars and canines (Figs 2-9 and 2-10). This is especially true in periodontal patients who have previously experienced recession. Careful recommendations and frequent monitoring of technique are critical for this type of patient.

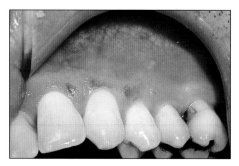

Fig 2-7. Clinical example of acute soft tissue trauma to the facial side of maxillary left teeth. The marginal gingiva is abraded and reddened.

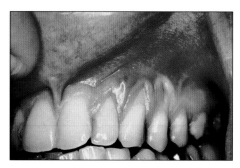

Fig 2-8. Clefting and recession observed with chronic soft tissue trauma created with a toothbrush.

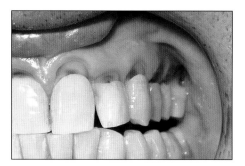

Fig 2-9. Facial side of left maxillary teeth with severe tooth abrasion created by toothbrushing trauma. Note that the damage is most severe at the cementoenamel junction and apical to it on the softer root surface.

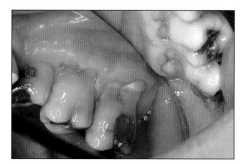

Fig 2-10. Severe abrasion caused by a toothbrush on a maxillary first and second molar. On these multirooted teeth, the recession has exposed the facial furcation.

When toothbrushing is complete and the accessible tooth surfaces and adjacent soft tissues are plaque-free, patient efforts can be directed toward other plaque-retaining structures. Reducing the bacterial load of the mouth may aid in reducing plaque growth on teeth. The tongue is one such structure that retains plaque and requires brushing. The patient is instructed to use firm, overlapping scrub-type strokes, starting at the back of the tongue and moving toward the tip, to remove plaque and debris. The gag reflex may determine how far back on the tongue a patient can brush, but the individual should be encouraged to thoroughly brush the entire surface.

Other areas that are often forgotten are the edentulous ridge and palatal tissue under a maxillary partial or complete denture. These areas also retain plaque. This plaque, an etiologic factor in the development of denture stomatitis, inflammatory papillary hyperplasia, chronic candidiasis, and offensive odors, must be removed. Removal is accomplished by brushing those areas with a soft toothbrush to remove the plaque and debris.

Interdental Cleansing

Although some cleaning of interdental areas is possible with a toothbrush, it is generally accepted that effective plaque removal is not accomplished with a toothbrush alone, since it is impossible to get the toothbrush bristles completely into the interdental region.[4] Several different types of devices have been developed to assist interdental plaque removal. Before recommending one of these devices, the clinician must evaluate the interdental region. This evaluation must consider such factors as: *1)* How well does the patient's toothbrushing method remove plaque from the interdental area? *2)* How much manual dexterity does the patient have for manipulating interdental cleaning aids? *3)* What contributing factors, such as anatomic variations, bridges, implants, orthodontics appliances, removable appliances or other restorations, are present that may make interdental cleansing more difficult? *4)* How crowded are the teeth, and is there evidence of demineralization or interproximal decay? and *5)* What is the size and shape of the interdental space—is the interdental papillae inflamed and bulbous, or is it blunted, cratered, or reduced in height?

After evaluating these factors, the clinician can individualize the recommendations made to the patient to aid in effective plaque removal. Adjustments in the suggested regimen are made as these factors change or are re-evaluated.

Anatomy of the interdental area is a major factor in the initiation and control of periodontal disease, as well as in the selection of an interdental cleaning device. Proper cleaning of the interdental area is therefore critical, since this area is most susceptible to the initiation of periodontal disease.[5]

Interdental Devices

Dental Floss

Dental floss is the most consistently and widely recommended interdental cleaning aid. Various types of floss are available, ranging from waxed to unwaxed, round to flat to spongy, and in different sizes, flavors, and colors. Despite the assortment available and its wide recommendation, studies show that only about 18% of adults use floss regularly.

Although many clinicians may develop a preference for one type of floss, several studies have shown that there are no differences in the cleaning potential of different types of floss. A study by Smith and associates evaluated the cleaning efficiency of four different types of floss on different tooth surfaces.[6] No significant difference was found between the different types of floss on smooth tooth and root surfaces, although waxed floss was found to be more effective on rough surfaces. Patient preference should ultimately determine the choice of which type of floss to use.

Dental floss is one of the few aids available that can be introduced into the gingival crevice and perform subgingival plaque removal. In healthy, properly contoured interproximal gingival tissues, dental floss can be correctly inserted 2 to 3.5 mm below the tip of the papillae without causing damage to the periodontal ligament or the gingiva. However, it is important to monitor carefully a patient's subgingival technique since detachment of the crevicular epithelium can occur. Other types of trauma have been associated with improper flossing technique (Figs 2-11 and 2-12). Placement of the floss and activation of the flossing motion are important since aggressive or uncontrolled movements or too much pressure can cause laceration of the tissue. Floss should not be snapped through the contact areas. Repeated trauma can result in soft tissue clefting (Fig 2-13). Controlled movements are essential to maintaining gingival health. Introduction and reinforcement of correct techniques require the clinician to allot adequate time to this phase of patient oral hygiene instruction.

The effectiveness of flossing is reduced in patients with a history of periodontitis and soft tissue recession resulting in open interdental regions. This is due to the presence of concavities, grooves, pits, and other variations in the root anatomy, particularly on the mesial surfaces of molars and premolars, resulting in regions of tooth surface inaccessible to the floss. Wong and Wade found that a type of floss with a section of expanded sponge (Superfloss by Oral B Laboratories, Inc.) designed to reach these more inaccessible areas was more effective in cleaning these regions than regular waxed dental floss (Fig 2-14). However, complete interproximal plaque removal was still not achieved. The Superfloss left

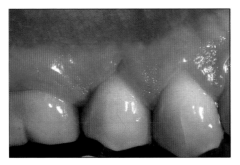

Fig 2-11. Gingival cleft in marginal tissue of the right maxillary second premolar. The cause of such unusual contours includes the patient's habitual hygiene procedures, so the patient should be asked to demonstrate the normal home care routine.

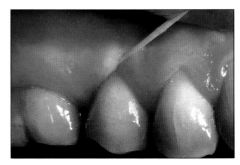

Fig 2-12. Observation of the patient's oral hygiene procedures demonstrates flossing trauma caused by an improper technique by the patient.

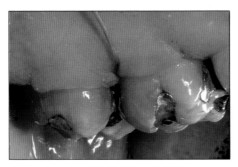

Fig 2-13. Clefting of the palatal tissue due to dental floss as a result of improper patient technique. In these cases the patient must be redirected in home care procedures and should demonstrate the altered technique to the therapist.

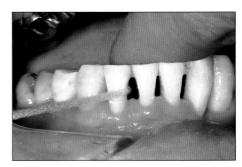

Fig 2-14. Expanded sponge floss in a patient with periodontal disease. The disease leaves wide embrasure spaces, and the sponge aids in plaque removal.

behind 49.9% of the plaque, and the waxed dental floss missed 54.7%.[7]

Even though dental floss has the ability to remove plaque in the interdental area, and it is frequently recommended by clinicians, routine use of dental floss by the public remains limited. This limited use may be due to: *1)* difficulty in mastering the technique; *2)* the time-consuming nature of the procedure; and *3)* damage to the interdental gingival tissues, causing discomfort.

Special patient and anatomic considerations may necessitate the adaptation of different techniques and/or devices for interproximal cleaning. Patients who have limited dexterity or who are unable to effectively master an efficient flossing technique may choose to use a floss holder. A slingshot-like device that stretches the floss between two pronged fingers can be used to work the floss between the contact areas of the teeth, scraping against the proximal tooth surface before being withdrawn (Fig 2-15). The patient must be advised to be careful when using a floss holder to avoid overly vigorous flossing, which may result in clefting of the tissue or gingival abrasion. This is more likely to occur with this type of device since wrapping the floss around the curved tooth contour is more difficult.

Other adaptations that may be used to increase the effectiveness of interdental cleansing include the use of knitting yarn or even gauze strips to clean more open, exposed tooth surfaces (Figs 2-16 and 2-17). Dental floss can also be used effectively to clean embrasures of crowns and bridges, between teeth that have been bonded or splinted and around fixed orthodontic appliances. Small plastic floss threaders, flexible needle-like devices with large eyelets, can be used to advance the floss under tight or closed contacts (Fig 2-18).

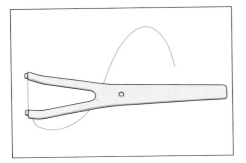

Fig 2-15. In a floss holder, dental floss is stretched between the two arms of a plastic fork.

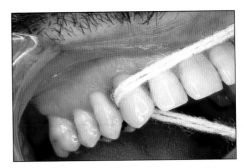

Fig 2-16. Single or multiple layers of knitting yarn can be used to remove plaque from enlarged embrasure spaces.

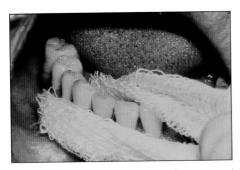

Fig 2-17. Strips of gauze can be cut and used to efficiently remove plaque from interproximal areas where access for placing the gauze is not a problem.

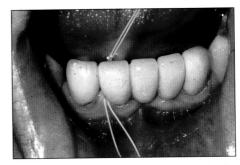

Fig 2-18. Floss threaders are used to facilitate the placement of floss under fixed bridge work. These threaders have a loop to hold the dental floss and a stiff nylon needle-like end to direct it under the dental work.

Flossing Technique

Flossing can be done before or after brushing, depending on patient preference. Flossing correctly is a definite challenge and often a frustrating experience for patients attempting to master the technique. Patients are usually instructed to wind the floss around one or two fingers on each hand (usually the middle fingers), grasping the floss between thumbs and index fingers, with the distance between hands just enough to allow for manipulation of the floss between the teeth.

The floss is introduced into the contact area, and moved back and forth in a gentle sawing motion until it is through the contact. The floss is then pressed against the interproximal surface of one tooth so that it contacts that surface from buccal line angle to lingual line angle (Fig 2-19). As the floss is continually applied to the interproximal surface it is moved up and down, scraping off the plaque. The extent of the downward motion of the floss is determined by resistance of the gingival tissue. Once resistance is felt, the floss should not be forced further into the crevice. The floss is then moved over the papillae to the adjacent tooth surface, and the scraping motion repeated (Fig 2-20). The floss is removed by drawing it back through the contact.

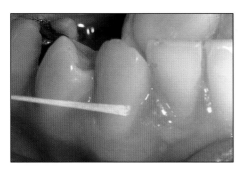

Fig 2-19. The correct placement of dental floss on the mesial aspect of the mandibular right canine. Note the subgingival placement due to the need to adapt the floss to the contours of the tooth.

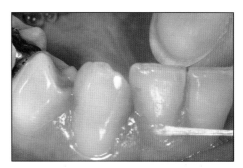

Fig 2-20. Before the floss is removed from the contact point, the floss is adapted to the adjacent tooth (right distal mandibular lateral incisor) and moved apically to cleanse the gingival sulcus of plaque.

Although dental flossing has been shown to be relatively effective in removing interdental plaque, it is a procedure that is technique sensitive. Careful monitoring and adjustment of this technique is essential for effective long-term use of dental floss.

Interdental Brushes

In patients with exposed interdental root surfaces, plaque removal with dental floss may be more difficult or less effective. Interdental brushes have been designed to alleviate the difficulties of interproximal plaque removal in these situations. These brushes consist of nylon filaments, twisted onto a wire to form a tapered (Christmas tree) or nontapered (bottle-neck) shape (Fig 2-21). Filaments extend from this coated wire at right angles, forming a circular shape that, when pushed into the interdental space, distort to more fully contact the root surface and reach regions inaccessible to floss (Figs 2-22 and 2-23). Various brush sizes and handle designs are available and may be tailored to meet the patient's needs.

In addition to these exposed root surfaces with anatomic variations and open interdental spaces, interdental brushes can be used to clean exposed furcation areas that are difficult to reach with other devices. Other regions that may benefit from cleaning with an interdental brush are under pontics, bridge embrasures, and fixed orthodontic appliances (Fig 2-24). Recent changes in the construction of the brush and the coating of the metal core with nylon make this device useful in implant maintenance.

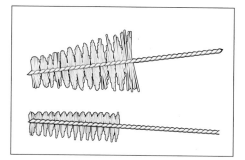

Fig 2-21. Interproximal brushes come in several varieties, including the Christmas-tree shaped style and the bottle-brush design. These brushes are available with plastic coating over the wire stems to help prevent damage to dental implants.

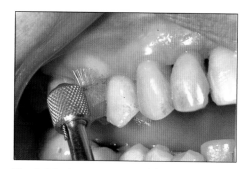

Fig 2-22. An interproximal brush is used to clean the embrasure of periodontally involved teeth from the facial side.

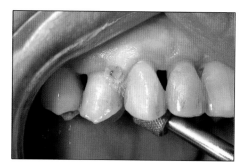

Fig 2-23. The opening to the tooth embrasures is generally larger from the lingual side, emphasizing the need for interproximal brush placement from that side of the teeth.

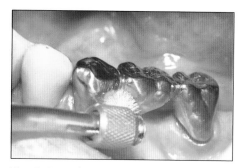

Fig 2-24. Placement of an interdental brush under the mesial aspect of the pontic on a three-unit, all-gold fixed prosthesis. Note that the design of the pontic allows easy access for the brush.

Single-Tufted Brushes

A single-tufted brush has proved to be useful in those regions not easily reached with other devices. Examples of such regions include irregular gingival margins around migrated or malposed teeth, lingual and palatal tissues that elicit a gag reflex with a full-size toothbrush, distal areas of the most posterior molars, orthodontic appliances, pontics, and precision attachments associated with crown and bridge or implant abutments (Figs 2-25 and 2-26). These special circumstances are often only identified after careful patient evaluation. These efforts again underscore the need for a long-term strategy in patient education that is flexible enough to meet the patient's changing needs.

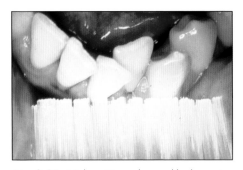

Fig 2-25. Malpositioned mandibular anterior teeth prevent access of conventional toothbrush bristles to the facial marginal tissue on the left mandibular central incisor.

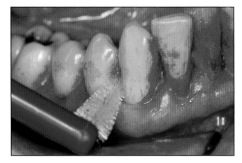

Fig 2-26. Lack of sufficient embrasure space precludes the use of an interproximal brush in the teeth stained with disclosing solution. This can be an important educational experience for the patient who needs to be motivated and educated with visual aids on the efficacy of plaque removal.

Other Mechanical Aids

A variety of other mechanical plaque removal devices are available (Fig 2-27). These are particularly helpful for the patient with open interdental embrasures to more effectively clean between the teeth and in exposed furcation areas.

Interdental stimulators are devices that have conical- or pyramidal-shaped tips of rubber or plastic and are attached to or inserted into a separate handle or a toothbrush handle (Fig 2-28). Firm application of these devices to interdental areas, using five to ten strokes per embrasure space with varying angulations, removes food debris and plaque. They can also be used to aid plaque removal in exposed furcation areas. Repeated use in conjunction with effective plaque removal leads to a more open interdental embrasure space, which the patient may find less difficult to effectively clean.

Dental woodsticks have a long history of use in tooth cleaning and have been extensively advocated by some clinicians for interdental cleaning. As in the case of interdental stimulators and brushes, they can be used alone or inserted into handles (Figs 2-29 and 2-30). Basswood or balsa woodsticks that are triangular or wedge-shaped to more effectively fit the interdental space are available. These should be moistened prior to use and applied with the broad, flat surface toward the gingiva. Once the woodstick has been introduced into the interdental embrasure space, it should be applied with an in-and-out type stroke with varying angles of application. Stabilization of movements is achieved through use of an extraoral or intraoral fulcrum or finger rest.

Many patients prefer to use toothpicks for interdental plaque removal. Toothpicks are available in many shapes and sizes and some are flavored. Round toothpicks, following careful instruction, can be used interproximally, in furcation areas and along the gingival margin. Handles, such as the Perio-Aid, make manipulation easier and help the patient reach more posterior or lingual areas (Fig 2-31). Patient

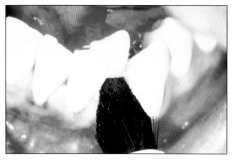

Fig 2-27. A specially designed tapered brush used to reach specific tooth or implant surfaces not accessible with conventional brushes.

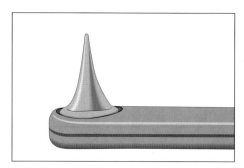

Fig 2-28. A conical-shaped rubber tip on the end of a toothbrush is used to help remove food debris and plaque.

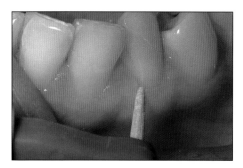

Fig 2-29. A rounded toothpick in a holder is used to clean plaque from the marginal gingiva.

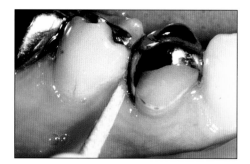

Fig 2-30. Dental woodsticks can be used to remove plaque from interproximal spaces.

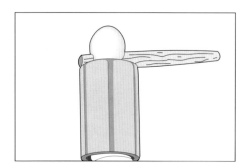

Fig 2-31. A device designed to hold toothpicks can aid in the placement of the toothpick tip.

preference and need should be the guide for the clinician in choosing the most appropriate toothpick.

An additional use of dental woodsticks is the application of desensitizing toothpaste or gel in exposed or receded cervical areas. Desensitization is often essential in achieving patient compliance for effective plaque removal.

Irrigators

Oral irrigators, developed early in the 1960s, originally received questionable reviews due to their demonstrated effectiveness against gingivitis but not plaque, and the fact that their primary benefit was seen as removal of food debris. Thinking at that time involved the application of the non-specific plaque hypothesis and the need to reduce plaque quantity to achieve tissue health. As scientific technology has advanced and the multifaceted character of periodontal diseases has been investigated, the benefits of oral irrigation have been reconsidered. This is particularly the case when one considers that the previously discussed mechanical devices have limited access to the subgingival space and the plaque that is present there.

Supragingival irrigation, using a standard jet tip, may deliver an irrigant approximately one-half the depth of a shallow pocket, allowing the patient to influence the subgingival environment (Figs 2-32 to 2-34). Patients should be instructed to place the tip at a 90-degree angle to the long axis of the tooth (not aimed directly into the crevice) and start at low pressure. The tip should be slowly moved along the gingival margin, pausing 5 to 8 seconds at each interproximal region. Tips designed specifically for subgingival irrigation have been developed that increase the penetration of the irrigant into the crevice. With the addition of antimicrobial or antiplaque agents, irrigators may now be able to reduce or inhibit plaque

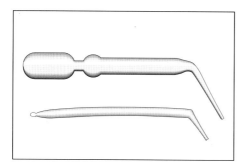

Fig 2-32. Subgingival irrigation devices are used to deliver liquids to the gingival sulcus.

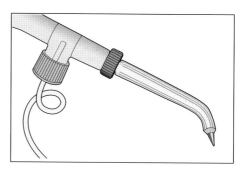

Fig 2-33. Another subgingival irrigation device. The tip of the instrument is shorter, but the device can be attached to a large reservoir of liquid.

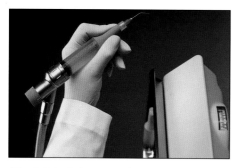

Fig 2-34. Subgingival irrigation devices are also manufactured for use by the professional to administer liquids into the gingival sulci.

as well as gingivitis. However, due to the limited penetration of agents, it does not appear that irrigation is able to remove or detoxify all subgingival plaque. Professional scaling and root planing is required to reach and remove subgingival plaque in moderate-to-deep periodontal pockets.

Care must be taken when recommending an oral irrigator or any adjunctive aid for patients at risk for subacute bacterial endocarditis or those with acute conditions such as acute necrotizing ulcerative gingivitis or a periodontal abscess.

Abrasives

Dentifrices are generally used in combination with tooth-brushing for the purpose of aiding in plaque removal and delivering agents to the tooth surface for therapeutic or preventive action. Generally it is considered that the therapeutic benefits of dentifrices outweigh the cosmetic benefits. Typical dentifrice ingredients include detergents, abrasives, binders, humectants, and water.

Of all the ingredients, the abrasives receive the most attention perhaps because of the potential for enamel and dentin abrasion. However, abrasives are included in the dentifrice formulations to provide for removal and prevention of the staining of the protein pellicle that forms on the tooth surface.

The most commonly used method for determining the abrasiveness of dentifrices is the radioactive dentin abrasion (RDA) technique. The RDA uses dentin of extracted, single rooted permanent human teeth as a substrate. The roots are cleaned, radiated, mounted in a slurry of dentifrice, and placed on a mechanical brushing machine. They are brushed with a medium-hard nylon filament toothbrush. The RDA value is determined by the amount of radioactivity removed from the root surface.

Research studies have demonstrated that even when a twofold difference exists in the RDA assay between dentifrices, there is no evidence of harmful enamel erosion. In 1982, basing its findings on this and similar studies, the American Dental Association established the safety level for dentifrice abrasiveness at an RDA value of 250. Currently, in the United States, most major dentifrices have an RDA value of 250 or less and are safe for public use.[8]

Dentifrice manufacturers have recognized the importance of dental calculus in the etiology of periodontal diseases and have focused efforts in recent years on chemical approaches to inhibit formation. Numerous calculus-control dentifrices are currently marketed. These agents contain a soluble pyrophosphate, zinc citrate, or triclosan as an active ingredient. In some cases, a copolymer is included in the formulation to invoke a synergistic effect. Each of these formulations has been shown to reduce the formation of supragingival calculus by 15% to 50% when used in a controlled clinical setting.[9-11] Few untoward side effects are reported during their use.

It is prudent to prescribe a calculus-control dentifrice for those individuals demonstrating a tendency to rapidly develop supragingival calculus in an attempt to reduce its rate of formation and potentially lengthen intervals between professional appointments.

Additional Devices

The recognition that dental calculus is an important component in the etiology of periodontal diseases, along with a general tendency of the public to want to control their own health care, has led entrepreneurs to develop calculus removal instruments designed to be used by the patient at home. These instruments are typically marketed by the local pharmacy or through the mail. They are advertised as being capable of safe and effective calculus removal.

Home-use calculus removal instruments are usually designed as a handle with some type of probe or blade attached. Patients are given instructions to carefully engage the deposit of calculus and physically break it up or dislodge it from the tooth surface. The instructions usually make the procedure sound very straightforward and relatively easy. In reality, the ability of a patient to maneuver a rigid instrument into a region of calculus deposition (typically on the lingual aspect of the lower anterior teeth or on the facial aspect of the maxillary molars) is extremely difficult. To then control the instrument so that adequate force is applied to the calculus deposit without risking slippage and trauma to the adjacent structures is virtually impossible.

These instruments must generally be considered unsafe, and patients must be educated that while home removal of bacterial plaque should be part of their daily regime, removal of dental calculus should be accomplished only by a professional dental therapist.

References

1. Gibson JA, Wade AB. Plaque removal by the Bass and roll brushing techniques. J Periodont 1977;18:456.
2. Adriaens PA, Seynhaeve TM, DeBoever JA. A morphologic and SEM investigation of 58 toothbrushes. Clin Prev Dent 1985;5:8-16.
3. MacGregor I, Rugg-Gunn A, Gordon P. Plaque levels in relation to the number of toothbrushing strokes in uninstructed English school children. J Periodont Res 1986;21:577.
4. Cumming BR, Löe H. Consistency of plaque distribution in individuals without special homecare instructions. J Periodont Res 1973;18:94.
5. Mauriello SM, Bader JD, et al. Effectiveness of three interproximal cleaning devices. J Clin Prev Dent 1987;3:18.

6. Smith BA, Collier CM, Caffesse RG. In vitro effectiveness in dental plaque removal. J Clin Periodontol 1986;13:211-216.

7. Wong C, Wade A. A comparative study of effectiveness in plaque removal by super floss and waxed dental floss. J Clin Periodontol 1985;12:788-791.

8. Pader M. Product components: therapeutic agents. In Pader M (ed): Oral Hygiene Products and Practice, vol 6. New York: Marcel Dekker, Inc; 1988.

9. Petrone M, Lobene RR, Harrison LB, Volpe A, Petrone DM. Clinical comparison of the anticalculus efficacy of three commercially available dentifrices. Clin Prev Dent 1991;13:18-21.

10. Scruggs RR, Stewart PW, Samuels MS, Stamm JW. Clinical evaluation of seven anticalculus dentifrice formulations. Clin Prev Dent 1991;13:23-27.

11. Schiff T, Cohen S, Volpe AR, Petrone ME. Effects of two fluoride dentifrices containing triclosan and a copolymer on calculus formation. Am J Dent 1990;3:543-550.

[3]

Mechanical Removal of Plaque and Calculus by the Professional

Mechanical Instrumentation

Mechanical removal of plaque with scalers is one of the most common methods of professional plaque removal. These instruments normally have straight-line, angular cutting edges. Scaling is defined as the removal of plaque, calculus, and their products from the tooth surface and can be either supragingival or subgingival. Short working strokes are usually used to accomplish plaque removal. Different instruments have been designed for different teeth and for the various surfaces on the teeth. The names of the instruments used in scaling procedures usually describe the shape and design of the instrument or the way in which the instrument is designed to be used. These instruments have been classified as chisels, hoes, sickles, files, and curettes. One of the most versatile and widely used instruments for plaque removal is the curette. The shape of the instrument allows for easy access to subgingival areas and is used with a pull-type stroke. The curette stroke can be lateral, circumferential, or coronal. The two cutting surfaces of the curette are formed by the lateral borders of the back of the blade meeting the face of the blade. The rounded tip of the blade forms the toe of the instrument. Only the cutting edge adjacent to the tooth surface is used in plaque removal procedures.

The two basic types of curettes are the universal curette and the area-specific curette. Universal curettes, such as the Columbia-McCall curette, have a blade that is at a 90-degree angle to the lower shank of the instrument and are used throughout the mouth and on any tooth surface. Area-specific curettes, such as the Gracey curettes, have an offset blade that is at a 70-degree angle to the lower shank of the instrument. The blade of these instruments is curved and only one of the cutting edges (the outside edge) is used.

Sickle scalers are also used commonly to remove plaque. The design and dimensions of the sickle scaler prohibit its use in subgingival areas. This instrument is commonly used to remove both plaque and large accumulations of calculus, particularly on the lingual sides of mandibular anterior teeth (Figs 3-1 to 3-3). Other mechanical instruments available, including chisels, hoes, and files, are predominantly used for calculus removal.

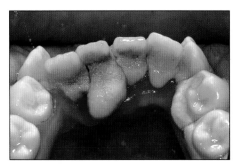

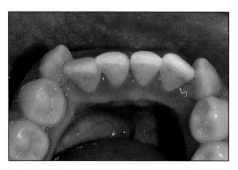

Fig 3-1. Gross accumulation of calculus on the lingual surfaces of the mandibular anterior teeth.

Fig 3-2. The same patient as seen in Fig 3-1 after calculus removal.

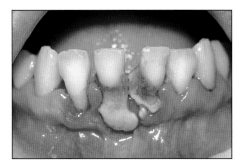

Fig 3-3. Another example of severe calculus accumulation. In this case the calculus has stains incorporated in the cemento-enamel junction area. Note the severe recession and intense gingival inflammation on the facial side of the mandibular left lateral incisor.

Electronic Instrumentation

Ultrasonic instrumentation is commonly used to remove plaque from the tooth surfaces (see Chapter 4). These instruments also remove calculus and stain from the tooth and are efficient in that a water spray is used as a coolant, which adds to the cleansing action of the instruments. These units are generally piezoelectric or magnetostrictive units, which deliver energy from an electrical power generator in the form of high-frequency vibrations. The vibrations of the removable tips disrupt the deposits from the tooth surface. The tips used in most ultrasonic instruments are available in many shapes and sizes. The handpiece and tip should be used with only very slight pressure since plaque is disrupted relatively easily with these instruments. In addition, surface changes in the tooth structure may occur with prolonged instrumentation or excessive force of the tip on the tooth surface.

Abrasives

Following professional plaque removal by mechanical and/or electronic instrumentation, the tooth surfaces are cleaned by polishing with an abrasive. The polishing is normally accomplished with a slow speed handpiece and a rubber cup. Many types of polishing pastes containing varying degrees of abrasiveness are commercially available. They are normally color-coded for convenience. Alternatively, a paste of flour of pumice may also be used. Some pastes contain sodium fluoride or stannous fluoride as a desensitizing agent. The purpose of polishing is to remove acquired pellicle and stains on the teeth.

Calculus Removal

Evaluation

Prior to initiating instrumentation procedures, it is imperative that the therapist identify the location and extent of calculus deposits. It is also important that careful evaluation of the tooth surfaces occur during the delivery of care to assure that as much calculus as possible is removed, although the ultimate success of therapy must be assessed by evaluation of the healing response of the periodontal tissue.

Direct visual evaluation of calculus deposits may be accomplished by when calculus is in a supragingival location or when an open approach to scaling/root planing is used. The use of a quality, front-surface intraoral mirror, properly warmed to alleviate fogging, and appropriate focusing of the dental operating light allow direct visualization of larger deposits of calculus. Adjunct forms of illumination, and the use of magnification, can be of great assistance when visually identifying the presence of smaller calculus deposits.

Detection of subgingival calculus deposits requires that the skills involved in tactile discrimination of root surface irregularities be developed to a high level and that an appropriate instrument is used. A variety of instruments are available for subgingival calculus detection (Fig 3-4). Dental explorers are effective in facilitating detection of calculus deposits because they are thin, have a sharp point providing good tactile discrimination, and come in a variety of unique shapes allowing the clinician to traverse many different clinical situations. Some explorers, such as those with a pigtail design, are very effective in evaluating interproximal tooth surfaces and furcation regions, but do not provide good access to deep areas, especially those on the facial or lingual surfaces of teeth. Other explorer shapes (no. 17 and no. 3) are more ideally suited to deeper pockets on flat root surfaces.

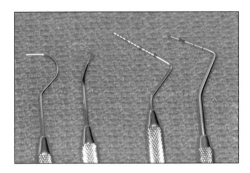

Fig 3-4. Instruments often used for calculus detection. From left to right are the conventional explorer, a "pig-tail" explorer, and two periodontal probes.

Some clinicians prefer to use a periodontal probe to detect calculus deposits, especially during an initial evaluation. The use of a probe for calculus detection allows the establishment of a very efficient diagnostic regime during which calculus detection can be accomplished without changing instruments at the same time probing depth and probing attachment level are being evaluated. However, the bluntness, straightness, and relative rigidity of the periodontal probe compromise its ability to detect small deposits of calculus in tortuous locations.

Regardless of the instrument chosen for calculus detection, it is imperative that a few basic principles be adhered to during subgingival calculus detection. The instrument should be grasped gently with the clinician's fingertips in contact with the handle. The tip of the instrument should be lightly guided across the root surface. The gentle grasp of the instrument with the fingertips and the light contact of the instrument tip with the tooth are imperative to allow maximal tactile discrimination. The instrument tip should be moved in an overlapping, multidirectional pattern to allow complete evaluation of all regions from all directions. With appropriate background training and experience, a clinician should be able to differentiate between calculus deposits, restorative surfaces and margins, structural defects of the tooth surface, root surface roughness, and regions of decalcification.

The clinician should attempt to keep the evaluated region dry during calculus detection. Saliva and other fluids may not only directly obstruct vision, but may also cause reflection of light that distorts and masks small deposits of calculus. A gentle, direct stream of air will usually be effective in keeping the region clear and dry. An airstream may also be helpful in situations where gingival tissues are inflamed. The tissue margins in these situation may be slightly retracted with a gentle airstream allowing direct visualization of calculus deposits in the subgingival region and easier adaptation of instruments.

Other aids may be of assistance in detecting larger subgingival calculus deposits, especially those in interproximal regions. Transillumination of the tissues, achieved by directing an intense light source through the tissues of the interproximal region, may demonstrate the presence of calculus. To be most effective, transillumination should be accomplished with a small, easily manipulated, intense light source. Fiberoptic lights may be used very effectively. The dental operating light should be shut off and the room lighting should be dimmed to allow maximal diagnostic differentiation with transillumination.

Subgingival interproximal calculus may be seen on standard bitewing or periapical radiographs. While concerns regarding repeated use of ionizing radiation preclude longitudinal use of dental radiographs to monitor calculus removal during therapy, radiographs obtained for diagnostic reasons should be analyzed very carefully to determine the extent and location of interproximal calculus.

Pain Control

Many clinicians use analgesia or local anesthetic techniques to enhance patient comfort during scaling and root planing procedures. These supplements are particularly helpful when procedures are time-consuming or are being performed for apprehensive patients.

Anesthesia

Topical Anesthesia. The use of a topical local anesthetic may be of some benefit during closed scaling and root planing procedures when the patient's soft tissues are sensitive. Before a topical local anesthetic is used throughout the mouth, it should be tested by applying a small dab to the oral mucosa and observing the region for several minutes to assure that a localized sensitivity reaction does not occur. If the patient exhibits no sensitivity to the anesthetic solution, a modest amount of gel-type anesthetic should be applied to the gingival margin with a cotton swab and gently worked beneath the gingival margin with a periodontal curette. The therapist must remember that topical local anesthesia only affects the soft tissues that come in contact with the anesthetic. It has no anesthetic effect on the root surface.

Local Anesthesia. Local block and infiltration anesthesia are indicated in all situations when an open approach for scaling and root planing is used and may be advantageous or even necessary in some patients, for extensive closed instrumentation. This is particularly true when the patient has extensive inflammatory periodontal disease and/or a relatively low tolerance for intraoral discomfort.

An appropriate guide for administering anesthesia for closed root planing procedures is to attain the same level of anesthesia needed for an intraoral surgical procedure. Nerve block anesthesia should be used whenever possible. In regions where block anesthesia is inconvenient, infiltration techniques to attain complete dental and soft tissue anesthesia should be used.

Analgesia

Oral Analgesics. Some clinicians have found that pre-appointment administration of oral analgesics is effective in raising the patient's threshold of discomfort during scaling and root planing procedures. Eight hundred milligrams ibuprofen 1 hour prior to a scaling/root planing appointment can be advantageous in raising the patient's tolerance for discomfort during instrumentation and reducing the degree of intraoral discomfort after treatment. Care must be taken when administering oral nonsteroidal analgesics so that potential toxicity and/or side effects are avoided.

Nitrous Oxide Analgesia. Nitrous oxide relative analgesia can be very helpful in raising the patient's tolerance level for discomfort during closed scaling and root planing procedures. When using nitrous oxide, the clinician must use a modern fail-safe analgesia machine with appropriate scavenger devices to minimize the accumulation of residual amounts of waste gases in the treatment room.

Intravenous Conscious Sedation. Intravenous conscious sedation may be a tremendous adjunct for some patients undergoing long or extensive scaling or root planing appointments. While use of intravenous sedation involves rather extensive preparation and monitoring and requires an appropriate recovery time, the time investment may be indicated in certain clinical situations. Intravenous conscious sedation, especially an approach with titrated benzodiazepine and narcotic combinations, produce an amnesiac state in the patient and allow rather long treatment sessions. Many clinicians prefer to deliver all scaling and root planing procedures at one appointment. This approach can be facilitated if the patient is sedated, comfortable, and relaxed throughout the session, which may take several hours.

Pre-instrumentation Rinsing

The oral cavity is populated by a host of bacteria and viruses. While most of these microbes may not be pathogenic in small numbers, the organized colonies associated with inflammatory periodontal diseases allow significant numbers of organisms to populate the areas to be instrumented with scaling and root planing procedures. A pre-instrumentation irrigation or rinse serves to reduce bacterial populations, thus assisting in protection against induced bacteremias during instrumentation or the development of excessive environmental contamination of the dental operatory.

Swabbing the gingival margin with 1% povidone-iodine has been suggested as a successful pre-instrumentation procedure as has a 1-minute rinse with chlorhexidine gluconate. It would appear that the chlorhexidine rinse would be the most successful in reducing bacterial populations prior to instrumentation procedures without undue side effects or complications. In addition, chlorhexidine has substantivity, allowing its antibacterial property to remain active after treatment.

Instrumentation

Hand/Mechanical Instruments

Scaling and root planing have traditionally been accomplished with the use of specially designed hand/mechanical instruments. These instruments are manufactured in a variety of shapes and sizes to allow maximal adaptation to the tooth surface and mechanical advantage to the therapist for the removal of calculus deposits. Each instrument is designed so that conscientious use will allow efficient calculus removal with minimal mechanical trauma to the root surface or crevicular soft tissue.

In general, scaling and root planing instruments are designed to have a working end, which incorporates the cutting blade(s), attached by a shank to the handle. Instruments may be single-ended with only one working end, or double-ended with two working ends. The design and angulation of the shank allows appropriate adaptation of the working end into the periodontal pocket while allowing the operator to maintain a comfortable, efficient grasp and ful-crum. Quality scaling and root planing instruments have a relatively light, balanced handle, with a thick, textured grip. The shank(s) may be rigidly secured into the handle or be removable with a screw-in design.

The cutting blades of a scaling and root planing instru-ment may be constructed of stainless steel, carbon steel, or tungsten carbide. Carbon steel retains a sharp edge longer than stainless steel, but corrodes easily during autoclave ster-ilization. Stainless steel scaling and root planing instruments with a layer of tungsten carbide have been introduced in an attempt to combine the best properties of each, but are rela-tively difficult to sharpen.

Zander[1] has described four modes by which calculus may attach to a root surface: *1)* by a dental cuticle; *2)* in irregulari-ties in the root surface; *3)* by penetration into cemental defects; or *4)* into resorption bays in the cementum and dentin. Three of the four mechanisms result in calculus embedded into the tooth structure, making removal difficult. Hand/mechanical instrumentation depends entirely on the working blade of the instrument, activated by the operator's fingers, to engage and mechanically sever the attachment of the calculus to the tooth. Instrument size and design are extremely important to allow effective and efficient instrumentation.

Hand/mechanical scaling and root planing instruments are classified into several groups depending on their shape and therapeutic role (Figs 3-5 and 3-6):

1. Scalers—Scalers have a sickle-shaped, pointed working end with an active cutting edge on each side of a triangular-shaped working face. Scalers are relatively rigid and heavy in construction and are designed for cleaving large deposits from the tooth surface (Fig 3-7). Their shape generally limits their use to supragingival regions (Fig 3-8). Positioning a scaler into the gingival crevice requires considerable tissue displace-ment and produces the potential that the instrument's pointed end may gouge the root surfaces or lacerate the soft tissue.

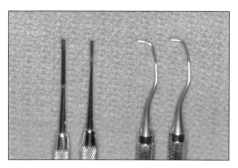

Fig 3-5. Hand instruments used to remove calculus. Note the variety of shapes and cutting surfaces. On the left are two chisels and on the right are two curettes.

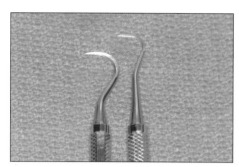

Fig 3-6. Hand instruments come in a variety of shapes and sizes. This picture illustrates differences in the shank of the instrument, that portion between the handle and the blade.

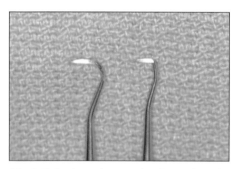

Fig 3-7. Both working ends of a scaler. The cutting edge is on both sides of the triangular-shaped working face.

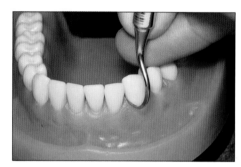

Fig 3-8. Placement of the curved end of the sickle scaler on the mesial aspect of the right mandibular canine. Note the position of the instrument handle and the use of the posterior teeth as a finger rest.

The relatively long, straight working edge of a scaler does not adapt well to concave/convex regions of the root surface, thus limiting the effectiveness of the scaler in root planing.

2. Chisels—Chisels are straight or slightly bent instruments designed to dislodge relatively heavy masses of supragingival calculus from the tooth in confined spaces. The chisel has a small cutting edge at the end of the instrument and is pushed between the calculus and the tooth surface to cleave the attachment. Although relatively limited in use because of the problems inherent in their use with a push stroke, the chisel may be the only hand/mechanical instrument capable of gaining access to regions such as the lingual aspect of the lower anterior teeth.

3. Hoe—The hoe is essentially a chisel with its terminal end bent at a 100-degree angle. This design allows the clinician to use the hoe within a pull stroke in confined regions. Because the hoe is relatively narrow and has sharp points at the lateral ends of its cutting edge, the therapist must be careful not to gouge the root surface when a hoe is being used. Hoes are most useful when used on flat tooth surfaces not accessible to curettes.

4. Files—Files consist of a round or oval base with multiple cutting edges lined up as a series of hoes. Files are relatively small and allow excellent access to subgingival regions. They are difficult to adapt to all curvatures of the tooth's surface and provide limited tactile sense. Files are also extremely difficult to sharpen.

5. Curettes—Curettes have been shown to be the most versatile and effective hand/mechanical scaling and root planing instrument. Curettes have a curved working end with a rounded back. The curette's tip is rounded, forming a toe, which prevents inadvertent gouging of the root surface or soft tissue trauma during instrumentation. Curettes are generally smaller and thinner than the other scaling and root planing instruments. Their size and rounded design allow the clinician to more easily maneuver the working end of the instrument into deep pockets or regions having difficult access.

Curettes are subgrouped according to their design. Universal curettes are generally designed to adapt to all tooth surfaces. Either cutting edge of the working end of a universal curette may be used in a pull stroke during instrumentation. These instruments are usually double-ended with each end a mirror image of the other. The blade of a universal curette is set at an angle of 90 degrees to the lower shank of the instrument, and the blade face is curved in only one direction. Universal curettes come in a variety of blade sizes, with larger blades designed to remove larger deposits of calculus from more accessible regions, and smaller sizes designed for the removal of smaller deposits from deeper, more restricted regions.

Location-specific curettes have specialized shapes that closely adapt to a particular tooth surface in a particular region of the mouth (Table). They are manufactured and distributed in complete sets so that the clinician can access all surfaces of all teeth throughout the mouth using the set. The most popular type of location-specific curettes are the Gracey instruments (Fig 3-9). These relatively small and delicate instruments have their cutting blade set at a 60- to 70-degree angle to the lower shank, allowing the outside edge of the instrument to be used in a pull or push stroke. The blade face of each Gracey curette is curved in two planes to allow more precise adaptation to specific sites. The configuration of the

Table. Applications of Gracey Curettes

Anterior teeth	Gracey 1–2, 3–4
Anterior and bicuspid teeth	Gracy 5–6
Posterior teeth, buccal and lingual surfaces	Gracey 7–8, 9–10
Posterior teeth, mesial surfaces	Gracey 11–12
Posterior teeth, distal surfaces	Gracey 13–14

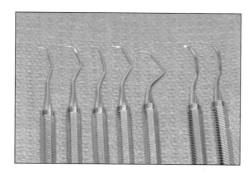

Fig 3-9. One set of location-specific curettes. These are generally sold as a set so the operator can treat all aspects of the dentition.

shank on Gracey instruments allows the clinician to maintain appropriate finger rests and fulcrums during instrumentation while maintaining the lower shank parallel to the tooth surface being instrumented. This characteristic allows the clinician to evaluate instrument position even when the working end is in a subgingival location.

Maximum effectiveness and efficiency while using hand/mechanical scaling and root planing instruments depend on precise control of the instrument by the therapist. Stable finger rests, with the instrument fulcrum position established to provide optimum mechanical advantage, are extremely important. Appropriate and carefully controlled finger, wrist, and arm movements allow the clinician to apply appropriate leverage and force to dislodge calculus and smooth the root surface without causing excessive muscular fatigue. The reader is referred to *Root Scaling and Planing*[2] for a specific discussion of appropriate instrument grasp, finger rest, and operator position during scaling and root planing procedures with hand/mechanical instruments. Regardless of the approach the clinician must remember to carefully evaluate each region prior to instrumentation. It has been documented that healthy sites will lose periodontal attachment if subjected to scaling and root planing. Scaling and root planing procedures should not be used in healthy sites.

Limitations of Hand/Mechanical Instrumentation

As discussed in Chapter 1, the success of scaling and root planing procedures depends on the ability of the therapist and the patient to reduce the level of etiologic factors below the threshold capable of initiating inflammatory disease in the host. Hand/mechanical instruments have specific limitations in some regions of the mouth that compromise achievement of this goal. Some of these limitations exist because of the inability of the clinician to appropriately insert and adapt the instrument while maintaining an appropriate fulcrum and mechanical advantage to allow the instrument to work effectively. This situation typically occurs during instrumentation of a deep pocket and furcations in the posterior region of the mouth.

More specific limitations for hand/mechanical instruments occur when the size of the instrument does not allow adequate access to a particular region. This may occur where root anatomy demonstrates grooves that are smaller than the working portion of the instrument or in regions of root proximity.

All hand/mechanical periodontal instruments must be of a size sufficient to ensure that the instrument has enough strength to withstand the forces that may be generated by the clinician. This strength is a function of appropriate metals and adequate size at the shank and working end.

Bower[3,4] evaluated the size of the working tip of a periodontal curette, usually considered to be the most delicate of scaling and root planing instruments, to the entrance diameter of the furcation region in multirooted teeth. The majority of entrances in maxillary molars (Fig 3-10) and mandibular molars (Fig 11) were smaller than the average width (1 mm) of a curette blade. Bower also evaluated the internal architecture of multirooted teeth and concluded that hand/mechanical instruments were ineffective in negotiating many of the internal intricacies that occur in the intrafurcal region.

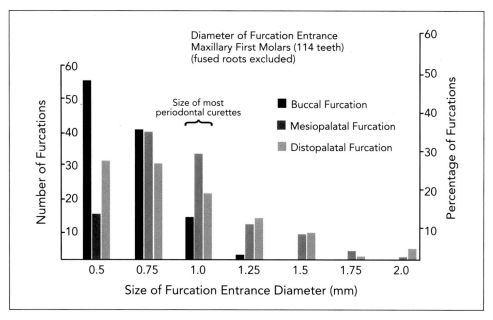

Fig 3-10. Distribution of furcation entrance diameter size expressed in millimeters for each of the three furcation entrances of maxillary first molar teeth.

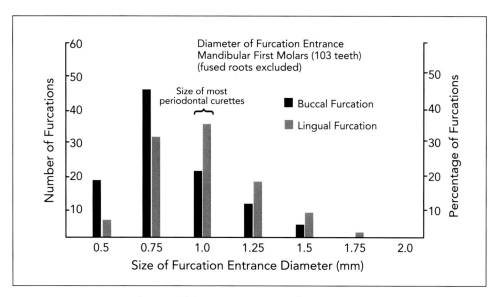

Fig 3-11. Distribution of furcation entrance diameter size expressed in millimeters for the two furcation entrances of mandibular first molar teeth. (Figures adapted from: Bower RC. Furcation morphology relative to periodontal treatment: furcation entrance architecture. J Periodontol 1979; January:23.

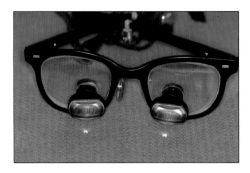

Fig 3-12. One example of available magnification lenses. These are custom-designed for the operator.

Adjuncts for Professional Calculus Removal

Magnification

Clinicians must have optimal vision during scaling and root planing procedures to assist identification of calculus deposits and adjust adaptation of instruments. Many have found that special eye wear that provides magnification is an invaluable aid. Some magnification aids may be custom designed (Fig 3-12). These magnifiers incorporate lenses with a specifically selected magnification ratio, focal length, and depth of field into a frame precisely fitted to the clinician. These magnifiers are comfortable and not fatiguing but they are relatively costly.

Other alternatives include adjustable lenses that may be modified to fit the clinician's needs and universal designs. The alternative approaches, while usually less costly, are typically bulkier and less convenient.

Illumination

While the dental operatory light may provide adequate illumination for many aspects of scaling and root planing procedures, consistent and effective illumination from the dental operatory light often requires multiple adjustments of both the light and the patient's head. There are also some situations when the therapist's or assistant's head may cause significant shadowing in the operating field. Many clinicians prefer the use of an auxiliary lighting source to supplement the dental operatory light during scaling and root planing procedures.

An incandescent head lamp affixed to the therapist's head provides a constant source of light directly to the region needed. However, these devices are costly, may be cumbersome, and restrict the therapist's movement because they require connection by a cord to a power source.

Fiberoptic illumination may be provided with a free-standing light wand or attachments to the dental mirror, retractor, or suction apparatus. The fiberoptic light provides a convenient, intense, cool light source directly to the area of interest and is very convenient for the dental assistant to use during scaling and root planing procedures.

Papillae Reflection

Many clinicians have identified clinical situations in which the desired outcome cannot be achieved with closed scaling and root planing, but traditional soft tissue reflection is not indicated. A modified surgical approach, involving the reflection of only the interproximal papillae, supplemented with fiberoptic illumination and transillumination, has been suggested as an alternative treatment approach.

Controlled clinical trials have shown that scaling and root planing with modified access approaches may be more effective in removing interproximal, subgingival calculus deposits than use of a totally closed procedure. One such procedure, with use of interpapillary incisions coupled with reflection, fiberoptic illumination, and air/water spray was found to be significantly more effective than a closed approach.[5,6] Results of this approach were similar regardless of whether hand/mechanical or powered instruments were used to complete the root instrumentation. While these studies do not allow one to conclude how much of the increased success was due to additional access provided by the interpapillary incision and how much was due to the features of the special retraction instrument, a treatment approach with minimal papillae reflection appears to be appropriate for individuals with moderate periodontitis primarily involving interproximal sites.

Root Sensitivity

Scaling and root planing procedures often expose a layer of dentin, especially in the region just apical to the cemento-enamel junction, where the cementum may be extremely thin. Exposed dentin may elicit thermal or tactile sensitivity in some patients. This sensitivity, resulting from exposure of dental tubules, is usually transitory in nature and a short-term annoyance. In some patients, however, root surface sensitivity can be a major concern.

All patients should be forewarned that root surface sensitivity to thermal change may occur following scaling and root planing procedures. This may be particularly noticeable when large deposits of long-standing supragingival calculus are removed. If a patient has experienced root surface sensitivity in the past or has sensitive teeth currently, he or she should be informed that the sensitivity is likely to increase for a short time after treatment. The patient should be reassured that sensitivity is usually temporary and procedures can be initiated, if necessary, to try and alleviate the problem.

Resolution of root surface sensitivity depends on several factors. Plaque must not be allowed to accumulate on sensitive tooth surfaces. Bacterial deposits will continue to irritate the dental tubules and not allow the accommodation process of the pulpal tissues to progress. It is thus imperative that the patient carefully clean the affected region. A coating of cavity varnish to provide a short-term obliteration of the outer surface of the tubules may assist in allowing the patient to initiate appropriate plaque removal procedures. A bactericidal mouthrinse may also be helpful during the first few days after treatment.

If sensitivity continues for more than a few days despite adequate plaque control, it is prudent to initiate the use of a potassium nitrate-based dentifrice or a fluoride gel. Both of these solutions work by providing a precipitant that obscures the dental tubules and, thus, reduces local stimulus. If sensitivity continues and is intolerable to the patient, more aggressive approaches, including the use of iontophoresis, may be indicated.

Scaling/Root Planing for Special Patients

Scaling and root planing procedures, regardless of the instruments used, have certain attributes that must be taken into consideration when providing care to patients with special systemic circumstances.

Cardiac Considerations

Scaling and root planing procedures have been shown to cause significant bacteremias.[7] While such a bacteremia is not a significant concern for most individuals, it is potentially life-threatening for patients with certain systemic conditions. A patient with a history of prosthetic heart valve replacement, congenital heart disease, valvular heart disease, or a subacute bacterial endocarditis are at risk for effective endocarditis from bacteremias of intraoral organisms. The medical history should precisely and accurately document the cardiac history of all dental patients. The histories of patients scheduled for procedures such as scaling and root planing, capable of producing systemic bacteremias, should be carefully reviewed. If any questions exist about the patient's risk for infective endocarditis, the cardiologist should be consulted. All patients at risk for infective endocarditis should receive prophylactic antibiotics according to the American Heart Association regimen prior to any scaling and root planing procedure.

Infectious Diseases

Care should be taken to avoid contamination of the airspace in the dental office during scaling and root planing procedures on individuals with systemic infections. Sonic and ultrasonic instrumentation, which creates significant aerosol, should not be used when there is a question regarding the potential of salivary contamination with pathologic bacteria or viruses.

References

1. Zander HA. The attachment of calculus to root surfaces. J Periodontol 1953;24:16-19.
2. Wasserman B. Root scaling and planing techniques. In Wasserman B (ed): Root Scaling and Planing: A Fundamental Therapy. Chicago: Quintessence Publishing Co, Inc; 1986:84-112.
3. Bower RC. Furcation morphology relative to periodontal treatment. Furcation entrance architecture. J Periodontol 1979;50:23-27.
4. Bower RC. Furcation morphology relative to periodontal treatment. Furcation root surface anatomy. J Periodontol 1979;50:366-374.
5. Miller CH. Cleaning, sterilization and disinfection: Basics of microbial killing for infection control. J Am Dent Assoc 1993; 124:48-56.
6. Wooten RK, Barata MC. Procedure specific infection control recommendations for dentistry. Comp Cont Educ Dent 1993;14:332-344.
7. Reinhardt RR, Bolton RW, Hlava G. Effect of nonsterile versus sterile water irrigation with ultrasonic scaling on postoperative bacteremia. J Periodontol 1982;53:96-100.

[4]

Powered Instruments

Powered instruments are assuming a rapidly increasing role in the removal of plaque and calculus (Fig 4-1). It has been predicted that modifications of the ultrasonic instruments may allow them to completely replace hand instruments (Fig 4-2).[1,2] This may sound like heresy to some since the curette has been the basic tool of root debridement for so long. Research, however, indicates that curettes have significant limitations (described in a previous chapter). In addition, debridement with a curette is a tedious, time-consuming, exacting procedure. Early reports indicate that the new, more narrow ultrasonic tips are easier to use and reach more deeply into periodontal pockets. They accomplish debridement faster than curettes and require no sharpening. Other powered instruments used for plaque and calculus removal include conventional ultrasonic and sonic inserts, air-polishing devices, and rotating burs. Lasers are being recommended for calculus and plaque removal, but in vitro studies suggest that they may create significant physical damage to the root surface.[3] Lasers, at present, are not recommended for root surface debridement.

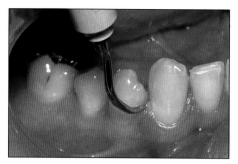

Fig 4-1. One clinical example of the tip of a powered instrument placed on the mesial aspect of the mandibular right first premolar.

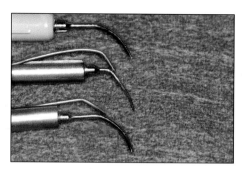

Fig 4-2. Powered tips that have been modified have been reported to facilitate debridement procedures.

Ultrasonic Instruments

Mechanism of Action

Ultrasonic scalers convert electrical energy into mechanical energy, resulting in a high-frequency vibration of the instrument tip. The conversion of energy is performed by either a magnetostrictive or piezoelectric transducer. Rate of vibration is 25,000 to 42,000 cycles per second with a vibration amplitude of 7 to 28 μm. Significant heat is produced in the conversion of energy. Water directed into the working area dissipates the heat and forms a fine spray from the energy release. The water spray helps to cleanse the work area and with the vibration energy may also have some bactericidal effects.[4] Calculus removal from the root surface requires contact of the tip against the calculus.

Indications and Limitations

Ultrasonic scalers have been used for many years to quickly and efficiently remove supragingival plaque and calculus, stain, and some subgingival calculus. Removal of these deposits is quicker than that with hand instruments, with less operator fatigue. Ultrasonic instruments are used during periodontal surgery to enhance the speed and completeness of root debridement. They are also useful in the treatment of ANUG and pericoronitis.

Conventional ultrasonic scalers have significant limitations, however. The working tips are bulky, making them difficult to use in deep periodontal pockets. Tactile sensitivity is also very limited because of the bulkiness of the tips. The water spray necessary to control heat production makes indirect vision with an intraoral mirror very difficult. Some patients dislike the noise production from the ultrasonic scaler; others experience root sensitivity during its use.

Ultrasonic devices are contraindicated for patients with older cardiac pacemakers because of the danger of interfering with the electrical mechanism of the pacemaker. Newer pacemaker designs with increased shielding may eliminate this concern. If the clinician is in doubt, he or she should consult with the patient's cardiologist. Patients with infectious diseases such as AIDS, tuberculosis, and hepatitis should be treated with great caution with ultrasonic devices because of aerosol production in the treatment room. A thirty-fold increase of airborne microorganisms in the treatment room is produced by ultrasonic scalers.[5]

Guidelines for Use

Ultrasonic scalers are safe and effective if used with the following recommendations:

1. Use enough water to avoid overheating the instrument and root surface.

2. Apply the side of the instrument (not the tip) to the root surface.

3. Move the tip continually in a back-and-forth brushlike stroke, avoiding heavy pressure.

4. Wear protective face mask and glasses during use.

5. Check completeness of deposit removal with an appropriate evaluation instrument.

6. Do not use ultrasonic scalers on patients with cardiac pacemakers without consultation with their cardiologist, and use with caution on patients with infectious diseases such as AIDS, tuberculosis, and hepatitis.

7. Flush water line for at least 2 minutes before use to decrease microbial contamination of the water lines and reservoir.

8. Ultrasonic scalers produce bacteremias similar to hand scaling so precautions are indicated for patients at risk for bacterial endocarditis.

9. Avoid bonded veneer and cemented cast restorations.

Effects on Teeth and Other Oral Tissues

The effects of ultrasonic scalers on enamel have not been studied extensively, but there is evidence from scanning electron microscopy that gouging of enamel occurs, especially at the cementoenamel junction. The extent of these gouges and their clinical significance are unknown.

Root smoothness following ultrasonic treatment has been extensively studied with profilometers and scanning electron microscopy. Hand instruments are commonly compared to ultrasonic scalers in these studies. The results are contradictory, making conclusions difficult. Roughened tooth surfaces have not been shown to create an increased risk for plaque accumulation. The amount of root structure removed by ultrasonic instruments is similar to that with hand instruments. Pulpal problems following ultrasonic treatment are rare, but the potential for significantly increased pulpal temperatures has been shown in extracted teeth.[6]

Diseased gingival tissues show rapid healing after ultrasonic treatment. Histologic sections obtained immediately after instrumentation show removal of crevicular epithelium and some connective tissue with localized regions of tissue coagulation. Ultrasonic scaling appears to enhance gingival healing after debridement with no evidence of unfavorable sequelae. No harmful effects of ultrasonic scalers have been reported when used near alveolar bone during periodontal surgery.

In summary, most evidence indicates that ultrasonic scalers are safe to use with the precautions outlined for periodontal therapy.

Comparison of Ultrasonics to Hand Instruments

Ultrasonic scalers have been compared extensively with hand instruments for scaling and root planing. Several reports indicate that ultrasonic scalers are as effective as hand instruments in removing subgingival calculus, plaque, and bacterial endotoxin from root surfaces; they are more effective in furcations and for stain removal. Ultrasonic instruments require less time for calculus removal, especially supragingival calculus. Healing of soft tissues occurs slightly faster after ultrasonic instrumentation than that after use of hand instruments.

Modified Ultrasonic Instruments

For many years, ultrasonic scalers were described as adjuncts to hand instruments in periodontal therapy. This idea is changing.

The curette has been an important tool of dentistry for almost a century. Research, however, indicates that it has significant limitations. Because of curette design, they cannot reach the base of deep periodontal pockets and are especially limited in furcations. Standard ultrasonic scalers, like curettes, are too bulky to reach into the confines of deep pockets.

When evaluating periodontal pocket depth, a periodontal probe is used because it is straight and narrow. A newer modified ultrasonic instrument is designed very much like a periodontal probe (Fig 4-3). It not only allows access to deep pockets, but allows movement necessary for debridement. There is a minimum of soft tissue displacement, and early reports indicate patient acceptance is very high because there is little pain or discomfort, which is often associated with conventional hand instruments and ultrasonic inserts.

A curette, by design, must be sharp and held at a critical angle with heavy pressure to be effective. Much time and effort is required to keep curettes sharp and their use can be very fatiguing. These restrictions do not apply to the modified ultrasonic instruments. No sharpening is necessary, they are less fatiguing because light, brushlike strokes are used, and the angle of the tip to the tooth is not critical for debridement.

Reports by Holbrook and Low[1] and Dragoo[2] strongly support the effectiveness of the modified ultrasonic instruments when compared to hand instruments. The investigation by Dragoo was a controlled study and found the new technique was easier to learn, easier to teach, most efficient in removing subgingival irritants, least damaging to the root, most effective for reaching the bottom of the pocket, and least exhausting for the operator when compared to the use of hand instruments.

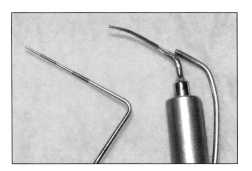

Fig 4-3. Some ultrasonic tips have been modified to mimic the periodontal probe.

Sonic Instruments

Sonic instruments (such as the Titan S) generally have been used in dentistry for the same applications as ultrasonic devices (such as the Cavitron). Most studies have shown no major differences in effectiveness between hand and sonic instruments or between sonic and ultrasonic instruments. The Table presents a summary of some basic functional differences between ultrasonic and sonic devices.

Sonic scalers offer some practical advantages over ultrasonic scalers. They can be directly attached to the air pressure outlet on dental units, thus making the equipment compact, inexpensive, and easy to sterilize. The multiple hose and connections necessary for the ultrasonic unit are eliminated. As noted in the Table, the sonic tip vibrates with less frequency but the tip travels a greater distance. Sonic scalers appear safe for the patient if the same precautions are followed as described for ultrasonic operation.

Table. Ultrasonic and Sonic Comparisons		
Parameter	Ultrasonic	Sonic
Frequency	25,000–42,000*	10,000–18,000*
Energy source	Electrical	Air-powered
Tip amplitude	7–28 μm	50–150 μm
Path of oscillation	Longitudinal	Elliptical

*Cycles per second.

Air Polishing Devices

Air-powered abrasive devices have the unique ability to remove plaque and stain from areas difficult to reach with other instruments, such as narrow interproximal embrasure surfaces, grooves, and crevices. These instruments have been used during the past decade to facilitate the removal of plaque and stain. They operate by directing a fine slurry of pressurized air, water, and abrasive particles (sodium bicarbonate) against the tooth surface. The suggested working tip pressure is 55 psi. Stain is removed up to three times faster with the air-powered abrasive devices than with a curette.[7] The use of these devices during periodontal surgery has been suggested to enhance complete root surface debridement, especially in furcations and root flutings.[8] The safety of air-powered instruments during periodontal surgery needs further study. They do not concentrate enough energy in one place to efficiently remove calculus, limiting their value during periodontal surgery.

Air polishing is safe to use on enamel unless the enamel has surface decalcification.[9] However, as little as 5 seconds of application on dentin or cementum can cause substantial loss of surface structure.[10] Tooth loss is related to time of spray application. Therefore, these devices should be used with great caution on root surfaces of patients receiving frequent recall treatment.

Air polishers may cause minimal marginal gingival trauma, which is usually undetectable in a few days. Pain complaints from patients during use of these instruments are rare.

An increase in roughness of dental restorations (including gold) with just a 5-second application of air polishing has been reported.[11] Composite resin restorations are especially vulnerable. Therefore, when using air polishing, root surfaces and dental restorations should be avoided.

The handpiece tip is kept 4 to 5 mm from the tooth surface and is directed away from the gingival sulcus. Emphysema has been reported following air polishing and, therefore, inflamed gingiva and areas where there is little or no attached gingiva should be avoided with these instruments.

In summary, air polishing appears to be safe and efficient if used for plaque and stain removal on enamel. It can cause damage if used carelessly on root surfaces, dental restorations, or in the vicinity of inflamed or unattached gingiva.

Rotating Instruments

Complex root morphology and tooth alignment often hamper complete root surface cleaning during periodontal surgery. Excellent supplements to hand and powered instruments are diamond burs with a fine grit of 15 μm.[12] The use of diamond burs in a low-speed handpiece with irrigation was found to be the most effective method of calculus removal from furcation areas.[13] Use of a fiberoptic handpiece and magnification with these burs further enhances completeness of debridement.

The use of these burs is especially important for calculus and plaque removal just before regenerative periodontal procedures. Histologic study of periodontally involved cementum reveals that microorganisms are commonly found penetrating 3 to 7 μm into cementum surfaces.[14] Leaving this portion of plaque or calculus may result in normal clinical healing of soft tissues but may interfere with periodontal regeneration.

A modified bur in a high-speed handpiece can also be used for root debridement (Fig 4-4).[15] One bur has a tapered hexagonal shape with six dull edges (Figs 4-5 to 4-8). The rotating edges dislodge calculus by vibrations rather than a cutting action. A polishing effect has been described similar to the action of a finishing bur. These burs remove some tooth structure, however, so they must be used with caution. A water spray must accompany their use.

Because of the problems and limitations of calculus and plaque removal in deep pockets and furcations, it is probable that powered instruments will assume an important role in accretion removal. They can be safe and effective if used with the precautions described.

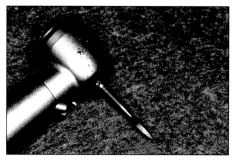

Fig 4-4. Root debridement can be accomplished with the use of specific burs in the high-speed handpiece.

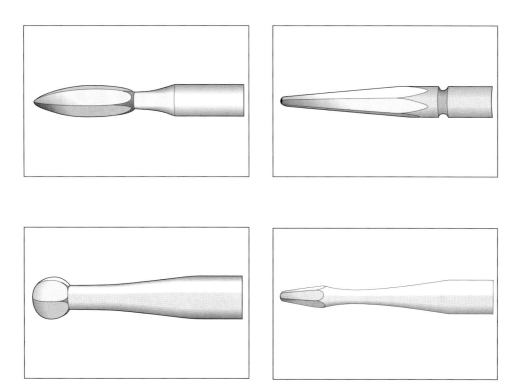

Figs 4-5 to 4-8. Burs used for root debridement. Different shapes are available to allow access to specific areas of teeth.

References

1. Holbrook T, Low S. Power-driven scaling and polishing instruments. In Clarke's Clinical Dentistry. Philadelphia: JB Lippincott Co; 1989.

2. Dragoo M. Clinical evaluation of hand and ultrasonic instruments on subgingival debridement. Part I. With unmodified and modified ultrasonic inserts. Int J Periodont Rest Dent 1992;12:311-323.

3. Cobb CM, McCawley TK, Killoy B. A preliminary study on the effects of the Nd:YAG laser on root surfaces and subgingival microflora in vivo. J Periodont 1992;63:701-707.

4. Baehni P, Thelo B, Chapuis B, Pernet O. Effects of ultrasonic and sonic scalers on dental plaque microflora in vitro and in vivo. J Clin Periodontol. 1992;19:455-457.

5. Larato DC, Ruskin PF, Martin A. Effect of an ultrasonic scaler on bacterial counts in air. J Periodont 1967;39:550.

6. Abrams H, Barkmeir W, Cooley R. Temperature changes in the pulp chamber produced by ultrasonic instrumentation. Gen Dent 1979;Sept/Oct:62-64.

7. Berkstein S, Ruff RL, McKinney JF, Killoy W. Supragingival root surface removal during maintenance procedures utilizing an air-powder abrasive system and hand scaling. An in vitro study. J Periodont 1987;58:327-330.

8. Horning GM, Cobb CM, Killoy WJ. Effect of an air-powder abrasive system on root surfaces in periodontal surgery. J Clin Periodontol 1987;14:213-220.

9. Boyde A. Air polishing effects on enamel, dentin, cement and bone. Br Dent J 1984;156:287.

10. Galloway SE, Pashley DH. Rate of removal of root structure by the use of the Prophy-Jet device. J Periodont. 1987;58:464-469.

11. Lubow RM, Cooley RL. Effect of air-powder abrasive instrument on restorative materials. J Prosthet Dent 1986;55:462-465.

12. Schwarz J-P, Guggenheim R, Duggelin M, Hefti AF, Ratertschak-Pluss EM, Rateitschak KH. The effectiveness of root debridement in open flap procedures by means of a comparison between hand instruments and diamond burs. A SEM study. J Clin Periodontol 1989;16:510-518.

13. Parashis AO, Anagnow-Vareltzides A, Demetriou N. Calculus removal from multirooted teeth with and without surgical access. (I). Efficacy on external and furcation surfaces in relation to probing depth. J Clin Periodontol 1993;20:63-68.

14. Daly CG, Seymour GJ, Kieser JB, Corbet EF. Histologic assessment of periodontally involved cementum. J Clin Periodontol 1982;9:266-274.

15. Ellman IA. Rotary ultrasonics for preventive periodontics. NY State Dent J 1962;28:404-410.

[5]

Maintenance of Instruments

Sharpening Rationale

A key to the effectiveness of hand/mechanical instrumentation is the sharpness of the instrument's cutting edge. Dull instruments tend to skip over calculus deposits rather than engaging at the interface between the root surface and the calculus and cleaving the deposit from the root surface. Dull instruments may also burnish smaller deposits of calculus, making them difficult to detect during evaluation.

A scaling/root planing instrument should be sufficiently sharp to allow the cutting edge to easily engage a relatively smooth material with moderate surface hardness. In the past, the thumbnail test was a popular and effective way to evaluate instrument sharpness. However, the use of rubber gloves during contemporary delivery of clinical care and during sterilization procedures does not allow the use of the thumbnail test as an evaluative aid. A moderately soft, acrylic cylinder (Fig 5-1) enables the clinician to achieve the same type of evaluation under today's infection control protocols.

The goal of instrument sharpening is to move or remove sufficient metal from the blade of an instrument to restore a fine line junction between the blade face and the blade's lateral surfaces. In most cases, this process is accomplished by sharpening the blade's lateral surfaces but, in some cases, sharpening of the face is required to maintain an appropriate instrument shape (Fig 5-2).

Sharpening is usually accomplished with a stone composed of silicone carbide (SC) or aluminum oxide (Al_2O_3). Usually a fine, mildly abrasive stone is most effective in maintaining an appropriate cutting edge on a periodontal instrument. These stones may be cylindrical in shape and mounted in a mandrel to be used following disinfection, but prior to sterilization, to reshape dull or misshapen instruments. The stones may also be flat and sterilizable, allowing use at chairside to sharpen instruments. Most clinicians prefer to use both approaches.

Many manufacturers of sharpening stones suggest the use of an oil-based lubricant during use. Since hand sharpening does not generate sufficient heat to require the coolant effect of lubrication, the main purpose of the lubricant is to prevent metal filings, removed from the instrument during

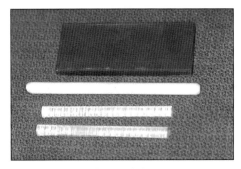

Fig 5-1. Flat and round sharpening stones (top) and acrylic cylinders (bottom) for testing for sharpness of instruments.

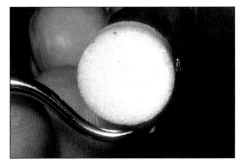

Fig 5-2. Sharpening an instrument on a round stone.

sharpening, from clogging the stone surface. Since stones with an oiled surface cannot be autoclaved, it is recommended that sharpening stones be used dry and that they be immersed in an ultrasonic cleaning bath prior to autoclaving to restore their abrasive surface.

Sharpening Techniques

The most effective method to use a flat sharpening stone at chairside is to stabilize the instrument on the edge of a sturdy work surface. Alternately, the instrument may be firmly grasped by the therapist who firmly braces their elbow and upper arm against the side of their body. With the instrument stabilized, the therapist may apply the sharpening stone to the lateral surfaces of the cutting blade at approximately a 110-degree angle with the blade face. The outline of the cutting edge should be followed as long strokes in a downward direction are applied starting at the blade portion closest to the shank and progressing toward the toe. The outline of the cutting edge that is followed will be relatively straight for scalers and universal curettes, but will require continuous change for limited access curettes. When sharpening procedures have modified the original shape of the instrument, it is appropriate to use a mounted or flat stone to consciously reshape the instrument to its original configuration.

An alternative to the chairside use of a flat stone for sharpening is the use of a tungsten carbide blade mounted in a steel handle (Nievert Whittler) (Fig 5-3). This instrument blade has one square edge and one rounded edge. When adapted to the blade face of a stainless steel instrument with sufficient pressure, it will move the metal of the instrument into a new edge configuration. The procedure, while effective, creates a small wire bur at the edge that then must be removed with a less aggressive stroke of the rounded edge of

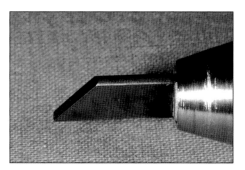

Fig 5-3. A sharpening tool made of tungsten carbide.

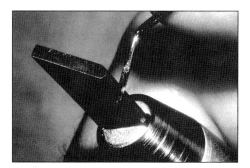

Fig 5-4. Instrument sharpening on the carbide tungsten blade.

the Whittler (Fig 5-4). While the Nievert Whittler is not an appropriate instrument for reshaping instruments or for major resharpening, it provides a convenient way to touch up instruments at chairside. Since the Nievert Whittler is constructed of metal, it may be autoclaved as part of the scaling and root planing instrument tray.

Care must be used with instruments that have been sharpened numerous times. The working tip may become very fragile and be subject to breakage during instrumentation procedures. If a tip should break during therapy, it must be clinically retrieved and identified or its location should be confirmed with radiography.

Sterilization

It is imperative that all practitioners providing periodontal care have an efficient system for instrument sterilization. Modern infection control procedures require that all reusable instruments being inserted into the oral cavity be sterilized prior to use.

Most scaling and root planing instruments are manufactured from stainless steel and should be autoclaved. Other methods of sterilization may be used, but stainless steel is susceptible to discoloration when exposed to certain chemicals. The manufacturer instructions for any chemical avoidance should be carefully followed.

Carbon steel scaling and root planing instruments require special handling since they are very susceptible to corrosion. If carbon steel instruments are autoclaved, a 1% solution of silver nitrite should be used to protect the metal from oxidation. Dry heat or chemical vapor sterilization is a better choice for carbon steel instruments. Regardless of the sterilization approach used, it is important to segregate stainless and carbon steel instruments throughout the sterilization process. Intermetal contact may facilitate corrosion.

Following a scaling and root planing procedure, all instruments should be deposited in a holding vessel containing an enzymatic cleaning solution. Instruments are much more easily cleaned if attached debris is not allowed to dry. Contaminated instruments should be confined to a specific area for processing to avoid any possible mixing with sterile instruments. Cleaning may be accomplished by hand scrubbing or by exposure to an ultrasonic bath. Although either approach can be effective, ultrasonic cleaning is much safer for the office personnel in that it avoids continuous grasping of contaminated instruments. Regardless of the cleaning method used, personal protective equipment (mask, eye wear, cover gown, and nitrile utility gloves) should be worn at all times to prevent occupational exposure.

Instruments should be transferred to an ultrasonic cleaning machine as soon as possible after use. The ultrasonic machine, containing a general purpose cleaning solution, should be activated for the time recommended by the machine's manufacturer (Fig 5-5). This will usually be between 6 and 12 minutes, depending on how the instruments are bundled. Sterilizable cassettes designed for periodontal instruments facilitate the management of instruments by containing them through the holding bath and cleaning, and into sterilization without direct handling of contaminated instruments (Fig 5-6).

Following cleaning, instruments should be rinsed with water and visually inspected for residual debris. If cleaning is not complete, instruments should be put through another cycle of the ultrasonic bath. When instruments are clean, they should be dried, placed in functional sets, and packaged, wrapped, and bagged appropriately for sterilization (Fig 5-7). The packaging material must be appropriate to withstand the high heat atmosphere of sterilization while allowing penetration of heat or steam to the instruments inside.

Packages placed in a steam autoclave should be subjected to an active steam cycle at 250°F for 20 to 30 minutes. A flash cycle of 3.5 to 5 minutes at 273°F may be used for un-wrapped items needed in emergency situations. Dry heat sterilization may be accomplished by placing the instrument package in a dry heat oven set at 320°F for 1 to 2 hours. All sterilization procedures should be carefully monitored. In addition to observing the gauges, dials, and printouts to assure that each sterilizer is functioning appropriately, chemical and biologic monitoring of effectiveness should be used.

Chemical monitoring involves the use of packages, tapes, or strips that change color after exposure to the appropriate temperature is achieved. They are used on the outside of instrument packages to indicate that the package has been processed through a sterilizing cycle. A more sophisticated chemical monitor, called an integrated indicator, changes color when a given temperature has been achieved for a specific time. Integrated indicators are placed inside instrument packages to assure that appropriate penetration has occurred.

Chemical indicators do not assure that conditions necessary to achieve sterilization have been achieved. To provide that assurance, biologic indicators must be used periodically to evaluate the efficiency of each sterilizer. A biologic indicator consists of a strip or vial containing highly resistant Bacillus species (Fig 5-8). A biologic indicator should be placed inside one of each type of instrument package used in the office and processed through each autoclave at least once a week. The most convenient approach to the use of biologic indicators is through a mail-in sterilizer monitoring system that supplies the biologic indicator, analyzes it, and provides a record of results.

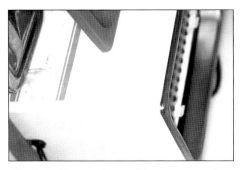

Fig 5-5. Ultrasonic machines are used to clean debris from instruments before sterilization procedures.

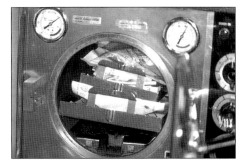

Fig 5-6. Sterilizing cassettes facilitate the cleaning of instruments since specific instruments used together can be grouped together.

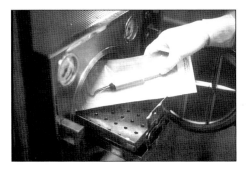

Fig 5-7. Instruments should be packaged appropriately for sterilization. Clear packages are useful for viewing previously sterilized instruments.

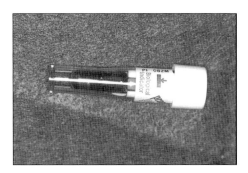

Fig 5-8. A biologic indicator for evaluating the sterilizing instrument.

[6]

Chemotherapeutic Removal of Plaque and Calculus

Mechanical plaque control procedures are the established mainstay for controlling dental disease. However, these efforts vary individually and depend on a number of influences that often result in the outcome being less than completely successful. In light of this, more recent research efforts have been directed at developing methods of enhancing plaque removal efforts.

As scientific advancements have confirmed the bacterial nature of plaque, antimicrobial agents have been developed and incorporated into therapeutic approaches. The inherent complications of long-term antibiotic use have directed efforts toward development of general antiseptics that may be useful in controlling the etiologic agents for infectious dental diseases. When evaluating antimicrobials, specific criteria are useful:

1. Does it reach the site?

2. Is it present in an adequate concentration?

3. Is it effective against target organisms?

4. Is it in the oral cavity long enough?

5. Does it have minimal/controllable side effects?[1]

There are presently several products on the market vying for attention. Of this group, two products are accepted by the American Dental Association (ADA) for the control of plaque and gingivitis: Peridex® (Procter & Gamble, Cincinnati OH 45201) and Listerine® (Warner Lambert Co, Morris Plains, NJ 07950).

Chlorhexidine

Chlorhexidine, a bis-guanide in a 0.2% concentration topical gel and rinse, has been used and studied extensively in Europe for decades. In 1986, a 0.12% concentration rinse was made available as a prescription agent in the United States. This antiplaque, antigingivitis agent has undergone extensive research, second in dentistry only to fluoride. Chlorhexidine appears to be the most effective agent available for the reduction of plaque and gingivitis. It has a broad spectrum of activity, yet development of resistance has not been shown. Short-term studies have demonstrated plaque and gingivitis reductions averaging 60%, while three long-term studies, examining over 700 subjects, reported plaque reductions averaging 55% and reductions in gingivitis of 45%.

The mechanism of action of chlorhexidine is tooth-directed and bacteria-directed. In relation to the tooth, chlorhexidine produces a reduction in pellicle formation and an alteration in bacterial retention and growth mechanisms, resulting in reduction of bacterial colonization on the tooth. An alteration in the bacterial cell wall, resulting from absorption of chlorhexidine, results in leakage of intracellular components and lysis. The key feature of chlorhexidine's effectiveness is its substantivity. Substantivity is the ability of an agent to be retained in the oral cavity and slowly released in its active form over an extended period of time. Retention in the oral cavity is related to the affinity of a positively charged agent to the negatively charged bacterial cell or tooth surface. Chlorhexidine is positively charged and has high substantivity.[2]

Adverse effects of chlorhexidine include tooth and composite staining the severity of which has been correlated to the patient's consumption of coffee, tea, and red wine as well as tobacco smoking. Alteration of taste following chlorhexidine use has also been noted. Chlorhexidine is marketed in the United States as Peridex (0.12% concentration mouthrinse, 11.6% alcohol, pH 5.5), with a recommended usage of twice daily. Adjunctive use of chlorhexidine has been shown to be effective not only in the management of plaque and gingivitis, but has also shown significant positive effects when used following intraoral surgical procedures, in a root caries prevention regimen, and as a subgingival irrigant. When used in a preventive program in conjunction with stannous fluoride, patients should be advised to use the fluoride product 30 minutes to 1 hour after rinsing with chlorhexidine to reduce a competitive interaction that could reduce the effectiveness of both agents.[3-6]

Essential Oils

Listerine (26.9% alcohol, pH 5.0) is a nonprescription phenolic compound containing the essential oils: thymol, menthol, eucalyptol, and methylsalicylate. Short-term studies have reported plaque and gingivitis reductions averaging 35% and long-term studies have shown an average plaque reduction of 25% and an average gingivitis reduction of 29%. Listerine is an uncharged compound and has low substantivity. The mechanism of action for this agent appears to be alteration of the bacterial cell wall and recommended usage is twice daily. Adverse effects of this agent are a burning sensation on the tongue and oral mucosa, and a bitter taste. Phenolic products are available over the counter and produce less stain than chlorhexidine.[5-9]

Non-ADA Approved Agents

Stannous Fluoride

Although fluoride's major benefits to dentistry have been to decrease the solubility of enamel to bacterial acids and enhance enamel remineralization, stannous fluoride has shown a secondary benefit of inhibiting microbial plaque accumulation. While short-term studies have demonstrated plaque reduction, statistically significant reductions and consistent results are lacking in long-term studies. The stannous ion itself may contribute to the mechanism of action of stannous fluoride, which is attributed to interference with bacterial biochemical synthesis, metabolism, and aggregation. It appears that stannous fluoride has moderate substantivity, with the 0.4% concentration being the most effective. Adverse effects are related to taste, a short shelf life, and the formation of black line stains on teeth. Stannous fluoride is most often available as an aqueous gel and suggested usage is one to two times daily. Stannous fluoride products have ADA acceptance for their anticaries ability, but this approval does not extend to or include their plaque or gingivitis reduction properties.[6-9]

Sanguinarine

An alkaloid extract from the bloodroot plant, sanguinarine (benzophenathradine) has, in short term studies, demonstrated some plaque and gingivitis reduction. It is available as Viadent dentifrice (pH 5.2) and mouthrinse (11.5% alcohol, pH 4.5). This formula contains 0.01% sanguinarine chloride. Long-term studies demonstrate effectiveness when subjects used both the mouthrinse and the dentifrice with plaque reductions of 17% to 42% and gingivitis reductions of 18% to 54%. The mechanism of action is proposed to be an alteration of bacterial cell attachment mechanisms and the degree of substantivity is unclear. Adverse effects include a burning sensation of the oral tissues. It is has not been approved by the ADA.[4-6,10]

Oxygenating Agents

Short-term studies of patients using oxygenating rinses yield inconsistent results and long-term studies show no benefits when compared with control subjects, for plaque or gingivitis reduction. A 1989 American Academy of Periodontology position paper cited numerous adverse effects relating to the use of hydrogen peroxide alone as well as a combination with salt and baking soda. These effects include tissue injury, delayed wound healing, potential carcinogenic or co-carcinogenic effects as well as *Candida albicans* overgrowth. Although most adverse effects are seen with respect to high concentrations and chronic use, clinicians need to consider the potential safety questions related to these products. There are currently no ADA-approved products.[6,11]

Prebrushing Rinse

Plax is the only agent currently available in this category. Results of controlled investigations have been inconsistent and unable to reproduce manufacturer-supported claims. Plax (7.5% alcohol) claims to enable the mechanical action of brushing and flossing to more easily remove plaque. The active ingredient is sodium benzoate and that combined with soaping agents may have a surfactant action on plaque. It is not ADA approved.[12,13]

Quaternary Ammonium Compounds

Short-term studies have shown an average plaque reduction of 35% following use of a quaternary ammonium compound with mixed gingivitis reduction results. Cetylpyridinium chloride (CPC) is the active ingredient in this group, known to consumers as Cepacol (0.05%) or Scope (0.045%). Scope also contains 0.005% domiphen bromide. The mechanism of CPC's action is related to increased permeability of the bacterial cell wall, decreased cell metabolism, and alteration in attachment of the bacteria to the tooth surface. Substantivity is low and adverse effects include tooth staining and a burning sensation of the oral tissues. The alcohol content of these products ranges from 14% to 18% and pH ranges from 5.5 to 6.5. Recommended usage is twice daily. They are not ADA approved for reduction of plaque or gingivitis.[14,15]

It is essential that both clinicians and patients recognize that no magic bullet exists to remove plaque. There currently exists no one procedure or agent that meets the stringent demand of clinicians, absolute plaque control, and that of patients, ease and negligible adverse effects. At present, it is necessary to selectively apply the cumulative effects of various mechanical and chemical modalities, individualized according to patient need. Appropriate therapeutic choices should be based on sound diagnostic criteria and be appropriately monitored. Adjustments based on disease process and characteristics, as well as on patient compliance, should be made as needed.

References

1. Schoenfeld S. USC Symposium: A critical view of antiplaque agents. AAP News, July/August 1987.

2. Kornman KS. The role of supragingival plaque in the prevention and treatment of periodontal diseases: A review of current concepts. J Periodont Res 1986;21:5-22.

3. Briner WW, Grossman E, Buchner RY, et al. Assessment of susceptability of plaque bacteria to chlorhexidine after 6 months oral use. J Periodont Res 1991;18:587-591.

4. Siegrist BE, Gusberti FA, Brecx MC, Weber H-P, Lang NP. Efficacy of supervised rinsing with chlorhexidine digluconate in comparison to phenolic and plant alkaloid compounds. J Periodont Res 1986;21:60-73.

5. Grossman E, Mechel AH, Isaacs RL, et al. A clinical comparison of antibacterial mouthrinses: Effects of chlorhexidine, phenolics, and sanguinarine on dental plaque and gingivitis. J Periodont 1989;60:435-440.

6. Otomo-Congel J. Over-the-counter and prescription mouthwashes—an update for the 1990's. Comp Cont Educ Dent 1992; 13:1086-1095.

7. Overholser CD, Meiller TF, Depaola LG, et al. Comparative effects of two chemotherapeutic mouthrinses on the development of supragingival dental plaque and gingivitis. J Clin Periodontol 1990;17:575-579.

8. Brecx M, Nekuschil L, Reichert B, et al. Efficacy of Listerine, Meridol, and chlorhexidine mouthrinses on plaque, gingivitis and plaque bacterial vitality. J Clin Periodontol 1990;17:292-297.

9. Comosci DA, Tinanoff N. Antibacterial determinents of stannous fluoride. J Dent Res 1984;63:1121-1125.

10. Hanna IJ, Johnson ID, LuJunec MM. Six month evaluation of sanguinarine products in orthodontic subjects (abstract 572). J Dent Res 1988;67:184.

11. American Academy of Periodontology. Hydrogen peroxide: Use or abuse (position paper). Chicago: AAP; 1989.

12. Grossman E. Effectiveness of a prebrushing mouthrinse under single-trial and home-use conditions. Clin Prev Dent 1988;10:3.

13. Beiswange BB, Mallatt ME, Mau MS, Katz BP. Plaque removal by a prebrushing rinse (abstract 1472). J Dent Res 1989;68.

14. Bemes GP, Roberts IW, Katz RV, et al. Effects of two cetylpyr-dinium chloride containing mouthwashes on bacterial plaque. J Periodontol 1976;47:419-422.

15. Compton FH, Beagrie GS. Inhibitory effect of benzelhonium and zinc chloride mouthrinses on human dental plaque and gingivitis. J Clin Periodontol 1975;2:33-43.

[7]

Implant Considerations

Dental implants have evolved from being termed experimental, or a last resort treatment, to being considered state-of-the-art treatment for patients who are fully or partially edentulous. However, for successful integration and retention of an implant, meticulous plaque control is critical. Before implant placement, patients must be assessed regarding their level of oral hygiene and be prepared for the strict measures necessary to minimize the potential risk of implant failure due to infection. It is important that the periodontium is healthy before implant therapy. Following implant placement, careful monitoring of the patient's level of oral hygiene and the status of peri-implant tissue is essential. Patients need reinforcement to maintain an exceptionally high level of oral hygiene, not just in the region adjacent to the implant, but in the whole mouth. Plaque in other areas may provide a seeding effect on the tissue surrounding the implant.[1,2]

Removal of plaque and calculus on dental implants is different than the procedures used for teeth. Innovative cleaning techniques are often required due to the nature of the suprastructure and substructure of implant restorations.

Implants and Oral Hygiene

Although the biologic attachment to an implant is absolutely different from that to a tooth, peri-implant oral hygiene measures do not differ significantly from nonimplant measures. A soft nylon-bristle toothbrush with an ADA approved toothpaste can be safely used to remove plaque from the implant abutment and superstructure. Access and tissue keratinization will determine the type (manual vs electric) and size of brush used. Interproximal plaque removal can be effectively performed with a nylon-coated interproximal brush, floss, or wooden toothpicks. Patients should use the most conservative approach warranted in each situation to effectively clean but not damage the implant surface. The long-term success of the implant depends on an intact implant surface and healthy tissue seal.

Plaque Removal on Implant Surfaces

Plaque must be removed from implant surfaces as well as tooth surfaces (Figs 7-1 and 7-2). Education in this area is one of the greatest challenges for the implant patient. The reason for this is that this treatment option is a relatively new procedure, it is expensive, and the surgeon often spends a great deal of time telling the patient not to chew or traumatize the implant site so that it will heal well and be successful. The patient may become sensitized to the fact that he or she will jeopardize the success of the implant if he or she touches or tries to clean the site. After integration, the therapist must then instruct the patient to change their behavior completely so that they are no longer afraid to perform oral hygiene procedures on the implant and restoration.

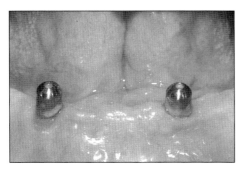

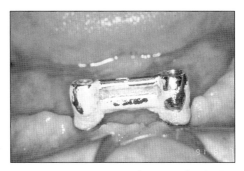

Fig 7-1. Plaque and calculus on the temporary healing abutments of two implants. Such accumulation is generally confined to supragingival areas.

Fig 7-2. Gross accumulations of calculus on the suprastructure connected to two implants that support an overdenture.

The additional challenge of plaque removal on implants involves access to the implant and substructure and the surface characteristics of the implant. Access to the implant and substructure is often very difficult due to the convergence from the implant diameter (usually 3 to 4 mm) to the crown. This situation is further often complicated by the use of a ridge-lap procedure in crown fabrication. These cases often require extremely difficult plaque removal procedures by the therapist as well as the patient. The use of removable restorations in this case is very advantageous (Figs 7-3 and 7-4). The surface characteristics of the implant also present difficulty with regard to plaque removal. In many cases, implants are used that have a rough and/or porous surface. These surfaces favor plaque retention and are extremely difficult to clean. Screw-type implants that have threads exposed present similar challenges.

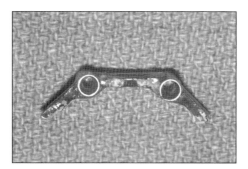

Fig 7-3. Calculus on the apical portion of an overdenture bar removed for evaluation and cleaning. Not all superstructures are removable (ie, screw-retained).

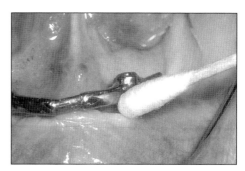

Fig 7-4. Cleaning around the implant and superstructure after an overdenture appliance has been removed. The cotton-tipped applicator is often dipped in chlorhexidine.

Many plaque-removal devices have been introduced that are specifically manufactured for implants and are designed to address the concerns previously listed. A concern about titanium implants is that the surface can be damaged easily. Titanium has a soft surface, and instrumentation can often leave a pitted or roughened area where plaque accumulation will occur more readily. For this reason, several manufacturers have designed titanium-tipped instruments, instruments made of gold, carbide, or plastic (Figs 7-5 to 7-7). Some of the instrument designs mimic scaling instruments, while others are designed to match the circular shape of most implants (Figs 7-8 to 7-13). The widespread use of implants coated with hydroxyapatite presents difficulties in plaque removal if the implant becomes exposed to the oral environment. It now appears that if the hydroxyapatite becomes exposed, it should be removed and the underlying titanium polished.[1] Removal of the hydroxyapatite can easily be performed with an ultrasonic scaling instrument. If threads are exposed, a diamond bur in a high-speed handpiece is used. In either case, copious irrigation should be used so heat is not generated through the implant.

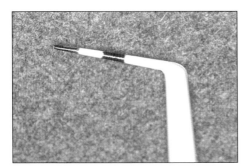 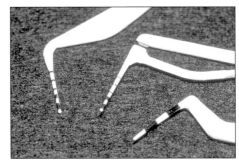

Figs 7-5 and 7-6. Plastic probes used around implants so the titanium or coated implant surface is not scratched. Different configurations and markings are available as well as a pressure-sensitive variety.

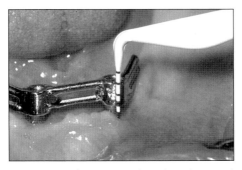

Fig 7-7. A plastic periodontal probe used around an implant. Fixed superstructures and attached restorations often make probing difficult or impossible.

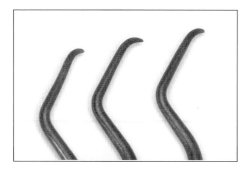 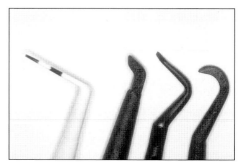

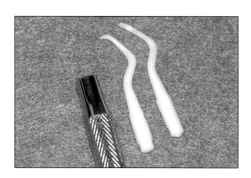 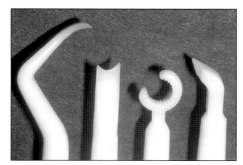

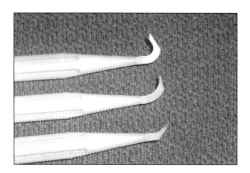

Figs 7-8 to 7-12. Instruments available for cleaning implants. Some instruments are designed to be similar to curettes and scalers while others are designed to adapt to the implant body.

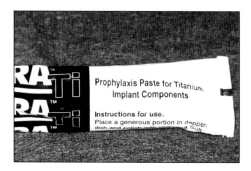

Fig 7-13. Prophylaxis paste specifically designed for implants is also available.

Many studies have been performed with use of different techniques to remove plaque, bacteria, or endotoxin from the implant surface.[3] In most of these studies, scanning electron microscopy is used to evaluate the quality of the surface after treatment. In most of these studies, the general conclusion is that the least abrasive method resulted in the least damage to the implant surface.[4] Therefore, from a clinical perspective, the therapist should begin with the least abrasive technique and evaluate if that has sufficiently removed plaque from the implant and restoration. If it has not been adequate, more abrasive techniques can be used. The least abrasive plaque removal method would likely be to use a thick floss or yarn and "shoe-shine" the implant post (Fig 7-14). This works well in areas that are difficult to reach such as the ridge-lapped restoration. Various brushes can also be used as a second approach to cleaning the implants and superstructures (Figs 7-15 to 7-17). Even though this is a procedure that should be performed by the patient, access is so often difficult that it may be necessary for the therapist to also use this procedure. If one can gain access, a rubber cup is usually effective for plaque removal. A next step would be to include a very fine polishing paste or a paste of tin oxide. Scalers, toothpicks, or other more

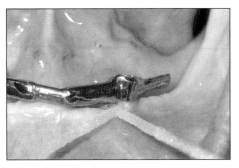

Fig 7-14. A relatively nonabrasive technique to remove plaque from implants and superstructures is to "shoe-shine" the structures with floss, yarn, or gauze. This is one of the few options for adequately reaching ridge-lap prosthesis.

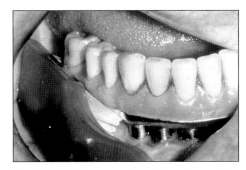

Fig 7-15. A conventional brush can be used to help remove plaque if the superstructure is sufficiently "high-water." These appliances are much easier to clean but can be nonesthetic and present speech problems.

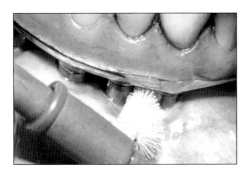

Fig 7-16. A proxabrush with nylon coating over the metal stem is usually an excellent aid to help clean under implant superstructures.

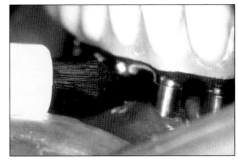

Fig 7-17. Specifically designed brushes used manually or in an electric appliance can facilitate cleaning. The single brush is often helpful for the patient to focus adequately on specific areas to clean.

abrasive techniques can be used if the more gentle techniques are not effective. Sonic-type instruments, prophyjets, or stainless steel instruments are not recommended. If the restoration is removable, cleaning is much easier as is the evaluation of the implant and restoration.

Patient education is extremely important, since patient compliance with an effective oral hygiene regimen is often very low. It is incumbent on the therapist to assure that plaque removal is being accomplished. Frequent appointments and customized instructions are very often required until the patient finds an effective means of plaque removal (Fig 7-18). Many options exist for the patient, including manual and electric toothbrushes, floss, yarn, gauze strips, shoe strings, rubber tips, proxabrushes, and rinses. Often, plastic patient mirrors can be used to aid in plaque removal procedures. The handles of these mirrors can be heated and bent to facilitate viewing of difficult-to-reach areas. Innovative approaches are often required by the patient and therapist to perform plaque removal on implants, abutments, and restorations.[5]

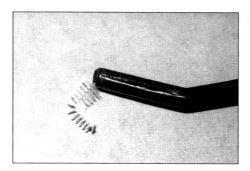

Fig 7-18. Modifications to conventional cleaning devices are sometimes required to help patients access certain aspects of the implant and superstructure.

References

1. Meffert RM. Treatment of the ailing, failing implant. Calif Dent Assoc J 1992;20:42.

2. Apse P, Ellen RP, Overall CM, Zarb GA. Microbiota and crevicular fluid collagenase activity in the osseointegrated dental implant sulcus: A comparison of sites in edentulous and partially edentulous patients. J Periodont Res 1989;24:96-105.

3. Zablotsky M, Meffert R, Mills O, Burgess A, Lancaster D. The macroscopic, microscopic and spectrometric effects of various chemotherapeutic agents on the plasma-sprayed hydroxyapatite-coated implant surface. Clin Oral Implant Res 1992;3:189.

4. Speelman JA, Collaert B, Klinge B. Evaluation of different methods to clean titanium abutments. Clin Oral Implant Res 1992;3:120.

5. Meffert RM, Langer B, Fritz ME. Dental implants: A review. J Periodont 1992;63:859-870.

Index

Illustrations indicated in *italics*.

A

Abrasion, *20*
Abrasive stones, 74, *74*
Abrasives, 35-36, 42
Abscess, periodontal, 35
Acrylic cylinder, 73, *74*
Aerosol, 59, 63
Air polishing devices, 68-69
    and emphysema, 69
    and enamel, 68-69
    gingival trauma, 69
    and tooth loss, 69
Airspace contamination, 59, 63
American Academy of Periodontology, 85
American Dental Association, 36, 82
Analgesia, 45, 46-47
Anesthetic techniques, 45, 46
    topical vs local, 46
Antimicrobials, 81

Antiseptics, 81
ANUG, and ultrasonic scalers, 63
Autoclaving instruments, 77

B

Bacillus species, 79
Bass technique, 17-18, *18*
Biologic indicator, 78-79, *79*
Brushing techniques, 17-18
    abrasion, *20*
    Bass technique, 17-18, *18*
    sequential, 19
    soft tissue trauma, *20*
    time spent brushing, 19
Burs, 69-71, *71*

C

Calculus
    accumulation, *41*
    attached to root surface, 49
    supragingival vs subgingival, 7
    visualized with stain, *4*
Calculus removal, *41*
    chemotherapeutic, 81-86
    evaluation, 43-45
    and implants, 89-98, *91, 92*
    and interdental cleansing, 21-32
    mechanical removal by patient, 13-37
    mechanical removal by professional, 39-60
    powered removal, 61-71
    rationale for, 1-11
    root planing. *See* Root planing
    scaling. *See* Scaling
Calculus removal instruments, 36-37
Candidiasis, chronic, 21
Carbon steel, sterilization of, 77
Cardiac considerations, 59, 63
Cavitron, 67

Cavity varnish, 58
Cementum, plaque penetrating, 8
Cepacol, 86
Cetylpyridinium chloride, 86
Chemical monitoring, 78
Chemotherapeutic removal, 81-86
    non-ADA approved agents, 84-86
Chisels, 39, *50*, 51
Chlorhexidine, 82-83
    adverse effects, 83
    substantivity of, 82-83
Chlorhexidine gluconate, 48
Clefting, soft tissue, *20, 24*
Coccoid, 5
Columbia McCall curette, 40
Copolymer, 36
Curettes, 39, *50*, 51-52, *53*
    area-specific vs universal, 40, 52, *53*
    limitations of, 54, 61, 66
Cyclosporin, *9*

D

Debridement, 61, 66, *70*, 70-71, *71*
    and ultrasonic scalers, 63
Dental explorers, 43, *44*
Dental floss. *See* Floss
Dental pellicle, 4, 42
Dental stains. *See* Staining
Dental woodsticks, 31, *32*
Dentifrices, 35, 58
Denture stomatitis, 21
Diamond burs, 69, 92
Dye. *See* Staining

E

Edentulous patients, 89
Edentulous ridge, 21

Emphysema, 69
Enamel, 64, 68-69
Essential oils, 83-84
Eucalyptol, 83

F

Fiberoptic handpiece, 69
Fiberoptic lights, 45, 56
Files, 39, 51
Floss, 22-28
    effectiveness in open interdental regions, 23
    flossing technique, *27*, 27-28
    incorrect use of, *24*
    with section of expanded sponge, 23, *24*
    use in gingival tissues, 23
    use for implants, 95, 97
Floss holder, 25, *26*
Floss threaders, 25
Furcation entrances, 54, *55*

G

Gag reflex, 21
Gauze strips, 25, *26*
Gingiva
    contours, *9*
    healthy vs nonhealthy, *3*
Gingivitis, *3*
    definition of, 1
    and plaque, 2
    ulcerative, 35
Gracey curettes, 40, 52-53

H

Hoes, 39, 51
Hydrogen peroxide, 85

I

Implants, 89-98
    coated with hydroxyapatite, 92
    instruments for cleaning, *94*
    and oral hygiene, 89, 90
Infectious disease, 59-60
Inflammatory papillary hyperplasia, 21
Instrument tips
    powered, *62*
    titanium-tipped instruments, 92
    ultrasonic, *67*
Instruments. *See also specific instruments*
    for cleaning implants, *94*
    electronic, 42
    maintenance of, 73-79
    mechanical, 48-54, *50*
    mechanical/hand limitations, 54
    powered, 61-71, *62*
    root planing, mechanical, 48-54, *50*
    scaling, mechanical, 39, 48-54, *50*
    shanks, *50*
    sharpening, 73-76
    sonic, 67-68
    sterilization of, 76-79, *79*
    titanium-tipped instruments, 92
    ultrasonic, 42
    ultrasonic vs hand instruments, 65
    ultrasonic vs sonic, 68
Integrated indicator, 78
Interdental brushes, 28, *29*
Interdental cleansing, 21-32
Interdental stimulators, 31
Interpapillary incisions, 57
Interproximal brushes, *29, 30*
Intravenous conscious sedation, 47
Iontophoresis, 58
Irrigation, 33-35, *34*, 92
    pre-instrumentation, 48
    subgingival irrigation, 33, *34*
    supragingival irrigation, 33

L

Lasers, 61
Lighting, 45, 56-57
Listerine, 82, 83

M

Magnification, 55, 69
Menthol, 83
Methylsalicylate, 83
Mirrors, 43, 97
Mouth rinses, 58
    staining from, 6

N

Necrotizing, acute, 35
Nievert Whittler, 75-76
Nitrous oxide analgesics, 47

O

Odor, offensive, removal of, 21
Oral analgesics, 46-47
Overdenture, *91, 92*
Oxygenating agents, 85

P

Pacemakers and ultrasonic scalers, 63
Packaging material, 78, *79*
Palatal tissue, 21
Papillae reflection, 57
Pellicle. *See* Dental pellicle
Pericoronitis, and ultrasonic scalers, 63
Peridex, 82, 83
Perio-Aid, 31

Periodontal disease
    chronic inflammatory, 11
    classification of, 1
    sequencing of therapy, 11
Periodontal pockets
    and furcations, 66
Periodontitis
    definition of, 1
    etiologic factors, 2
    and plaque, 2
Phenolic products, 84
Pig-tail dental explorers, 43, *44*
Plaque
    bacterial composition, 5
    formation, 4-5
    and gingivitis, 2
    penetrating cementum, *8*
    and periodontitis, 2
    significance of, 1-2
    on the tongue, 21
    visualized with stain, *4*, 13-14
Plaque disclosants, 14
Plaque removal
    chemotherapeutic, 81-86
    and implants, 89-98, *91, 92*
    importance of, 6
    and interdental cleansing, 21-32
    main areas of accumulation, 6
    mechanical removal by patient, 13-37
    mechanical removal by professional, 39-60
    powered removal, 61-71
    rationale for, 1-11
    root planing. *See* Root planing
    scaling. *See* Scaling
Plax, 85
Povidone-iodine rinsing, 48
Probes, 43, *44*, 66, *67, 93*
    plastic, *93*
Prophylaxis paste, *95*
Proxabrushes, *96*, 97
Pulpal problems, 64

Q

Quaternary ammonium compounds, 86

R

Radioactive dentin abrasion, 35-36
Radiographs, 45, 76
Recession, *20*
Ridge-lapped restoration, 95
Rinsing, 47-48
    chlorhexidine gluconate, 48
    povidone-iodine, 48
    prebrushing, 85-86
Root debridement. *See* Debridement
Root planing, 7-11, *8*, 35
    cardiac considerations, 59
    closed vs open, 9-11
    definition, 7
    infectious disease, 59-60
    instruments, 73
    mechanical instruments, 48-54
    pain control, 45-47
    therapeutic end, 8
Root, *8*
Root Scaling and Planing, 53
Root sensitivity, 57-58
Root smoothness, 64
Root surfaces, exposed interdental, 28
Rotating instruments, 69-71, *71*
Rubber cup for implants, 95
Rubber tips, 31, *32*, 97

S

Sanguinarine, 84-85
Scalers, 49, 50, 51. *See also* Sonic scalers; Ultrasonic scalers
Scaling, 7-11, 35
    cardiac considerations, 59
    closed vs open, 9-11

definition, 7, 39
infectious disease, 59-60
instruments, 73
mechanical instruments, 48-54
pain control, 45-47
supragingival vs subgingival, 9
therapeutic end, 8
Scope, 86
Sharpening instruments, 73-76
Sharpening stones, 74, *74*, 75
"Shoe-shine" technique, 95, *96*. *See also* Yarn
Sickle scaler, 40, *50*
Sickles, 39
Single-tufted brushes, 30, *30*
Soft tissue trauma, *20*
Sonic instruments, 67-68
vs ultrasonic, 68
Sonic scalers, 67
Staining, *4*, 5-6, 14, *30*
and abrasives to remove, 42
from chlorhexidine, 83
from mouth rinses, 6
Stainless steel, sterilization of, 77
Stannous fluoride, 84
Sterilization of instruments, 76-79, *79*
autoclaving instruments, 77
carbon steel, 77
intermetal contact, 77
packaging material, 78, *79*
stainless steel, 77
ultrasonic cleaning, 77, *79*
Sterilizing cassettes, 77-78, *79*
Streptococci, 5
Substantivity, definition of, 82-83
Superfloss, 23

T

Thymol, 83
Titanium implants, 92
Titanium-tipped instruments, 92

Titan S, 67
Tongue, and plaque, 21
Toothbrushes, 15-21. *See also* Brushing techniques
   conical rubber tips, 31, *32*, 97
   design, 15-16, *16*
   electric, 18
   end-tufted, *17*
   evaluation, 15
   flat plane of bristles, *16*
   and implants, 90
   interdental brushes, 28, *29*
   modified, *17*
   replacement, 16
   rippled bristle pattern, *16*
   single-tufted brushes, 30, *30*
   tapered, *32*
   using for implants, 95, *96*, 97, *97*
Toothpicks, 31, *32*
   handles for, 31, *32*
Triclosan, 36
Tungsten carbide blade, 75-76, *76*

U

Ultrasonic cleaning, 77, *79*
Ultrasonic instruments
   vs sonic, 68
Ultrasonic probe, 66, *67*
Ultrasonic scalers, 62-66, 92
   and ANUG, 63
   and debridement, 63
   effects on oral tissues, 64-65
   effects on teeth, 64-65
   guidelines for use, 63-64
   vs hand instruments, 65
   indications, 62-63
   limitations, 62-63
   mechanism of action, 62
   modified, 65-66
   and pacemakers, 63
   and pericoronitis, 63

W

Woodsticks, 31, *32*

Y

Yarn, 25, *26*
    using for implants, 95, *96*, 97